THE
FUNDAMENTAL CRISIS
IN PSYCHIATRY

THE
FUNDAMENTAL CRISIS
IN PSYCHIATRY

Unreliability of Diagnosis

By

KENNETH MARK COLBY, M.D.

and

JAMES E. SPAR, M.D.

The Neuropsychiatric Institute
University of California School of Medicine
at Los Angeles
Los Angeles, California

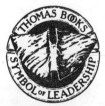

CHARLES C THOMAS • PUBLISHER
Springfield • Illinois • U.S.A.

Published and Distributed Throughout the World by

CHARLES C THOMAS • PUBLISHER
2600 South First Street
Springfield, Illinois, 62717, U.S.A.

© *1983 by* CHARLES C THOMAS • PUBLISHER

ISBN 0-398-04788-X

Library of Congress Catalog Card Number: 82-19206

Printed in the United States of America
CU-RX-1

Library of Congress Cataloging in Publication Data

Colby, Kenneth Mark.
    The fundamental crisis in psychiatry.

    Bibliography: p.
    Includes index.
    1. Psychology, Pathological--Diagnosis. 2. Psych-
iatry--Philosophy. 3. Diagnosis, Differential.
I. Spar, James E. II. Title. [DNLM: 1. Mental
disorders--Diagnosis. 2. Nomenclature. WM 141 C686f]
RC469.C64   1983   616.89'0075   82-19206
ISBN 0-398-04788-X

INTRODUCTION

THIS book addresses itself to what we take to be a crisis problem in modern psychiatry, that of diagnostic taxonomy. As illustrated in the literature to be quoted, there exist several schools of thought on its significance, its solubility, the desirability of finding its solution, and the solution itself. We have adopted a dialogue format with liberal footnotes to allow reasonable representation of several of these conflicting schools. The book should be taken slowly in small segments. It is not intended to be read straight through in one or two sittings. The issues are rich and profound. At times, the going is so thick that it should bring reading to a stop for the time being. The work is perhaps more re-readable than readable.

As the dialogues progress, the reader will find, as did the authors, that the problem under consideration is so fundamental that it ceases to be specific to psychiatry, or medicine, or even scientific-technological disciplines in general. Rather, the argument soon becomes concerned with three questions: (1) What are the entities that a particular theoretical or practical discipline recognizes as real? (2) How does one know when one of them has been encountered? (3) How can principles be articulated so that useful agreement on both of these questions can be reached by workers in that discipline? Undercutting the categories of ontology, epistemology, ideal and real, theoretical and empirical, the argument entails digression, repetition, ambiguity and redundancy, reflecting as it does the manner in which the issue was joined in the real-life experience of two concerned psychiatrists.

Like most real-life arguments, this one leads to no conclusive solutions. As Poincaré noted for mathematics, problems are not solved, they are only more or less solved. We delineate the crisis problem, introduce new problems, suggest some new vantage points and, we hope, demonstrate to the reader the difficulty with which conceptual and practical clarity of thinking is attainable in any field.

We are indebted to Flora Degen, for the heroic task of keeping this complex tome coherent through the course of continuous revisions, and to the scholarship of David Gordon for many corrections and emendations.

Kenneth Mark Colby
James E. Spar

SETTING

T HE time is the twelfth of Never. The place is anywhere people can talk without interruption, especially from a telephone. In the background there is a blackboard. The dialogue characters appear pairwise with a first party, the Inquirer (about whom little is known), discussing with various second parties the fundamental crisis of current psychiatry, namely, its diagnostic classification scheme. Each dialogue is overheard offstage by the other dialogue participants. In the finale, all participants gather together, and everyone gets to have his say with any of the others. Footnotes, comments, and references have been supplied by an almost omniscient Observer, not only to break the arduousness of following dialogue arguments, but also to provide sources of information for those interested in excursions into further detail.

CONTENTS

ix

THE
FUNDAMENTAL CRISIS
IN PSYCHIATRY

Dialogue I

THE YOUNG PSYCHIATRIST

O UR Inquirer first talks with a Young Psychiatrist who is finishing his residency and is about to enter private practice. He wears a beard and no tie.

Young
Psychiatrist: What do you mean "psychiatry is weak at its foundation"? Modern psychiatry has a solid basis in science.

Inquirer: Psychiatry itself is not a science; it is a type of technology, a craft, a practical art like medicine. We would like to raise it from a craft to a more intelligible technology. A scientist tries to understand how things in the world work. He searches for deep truth. A technologist is an interventionist who tries to get things within his reach to work for him in accordance with his purposes and values.[1] He is interested in rules of efficient practical action, and he is in a hurry to get useful results.

Perhaps so that they will be listened to by the public as scientists are, some psychiatrists like to talk about the "science" of psychiatry.[2] But psychiatrists are not scientists; they are craftsmen interested in successful action, not pure knowledge or deep truth. One

---

[1] The relevant distinctions between science and technology are made in Bunge, M.: *Scientific Research*, Vol. II (New York, Springer-Verlag, 1967, pp. 121-150) and, in regard to psychotherapy technology in psychiatry, in Colby, K. M.: Psychological treatment of mental disorders. In Sills, D. S. (Ed.): *International Encyclopedia of the Social Sciences*, Vol. 10 (New York, Macmillan and Free Press, 1968, p. 174). Some psychiatrists confuse the treatment of patients with a scientific study of treatment. Because a subject can be studied scientifically does not imply that the subject itself is scientific.

[2] Among some scientists, psychiatry stands in disrepute these days. For example, Gellner, a behavioral scientist, maintains " . . . the cognitively dubious practices in areas such as psychiatry willingly and eagerly assume the garb of science, and thus pay homage to the recognized paradigm of truth, as hypocrisy pays homage to virtue." In Gellner, E.: *Legitimation of Belief* (New York, Cambridge University Press, 1974, p. 193). Psychiatry may be in a crisis of confidence and not doing as well with its problems as it might, but diatribes do not make the problems (or the patients) go away.

could justifiably speak of "psychiatric sciences" referring to those sciences which contribute knowledge to psychiatric practice, just as the term *medical sciences* refers to physiology, biochemistry, and pathology. It is difficult for a technology to make progress when large gaps or weaknesses exist in its very foundations. A field must first notice, recognize, describe, and classify its objects of inquiry in an agreed-on vocabulary so that we know what is being talked about and so incoming students of the field can find out what it is that we are talking about.[3] Psychiatry is weak at its foundations because it does not adequately meet this core problem of taxonomy.

Young
Psychiatrist: Psychiatrists don't know what it is they are talking about?

Inquirer: When it comes to classifying our patients . . . no. The official classification scheme, found in the *Diagnostic and Statistical Manuals* of the American Psychiatric Association (DSM-II, DSM-III), is replete with vaguenesses, ambiguities, uncertainties, and plain errors.[4] I refer you to some recent literature.[5] As an example of what you will face in private practice, suppose I say I would like to refer a schizophrenic to you. What sort of patient do you imagine you would be seeing?

Young
Psychiatrist: A patient who is withdrawn, has hallucinations and perhaps delusions.

---

[3]This was succinctly put by Simpson in relation to biological taxonomy. In Simpson, G. *Principles of Animal Taxonomy* (New York, Columbia University Press, 1961).

[4]These manuals have been published by the American Psychiatric Association, *Diagnostic and Statistical Manual of the Mental Disorders* (DSM-II, 2nd ed., 1968; DSM-III, 3rd ed., Washington, D.C. 1980). In spite of their titles, there are no statistics in the manuals. They provide guidelines, however, for hospitals and clinics to collect statistics for classes of mental disorders.

[5]Panzetta, A. F.: Towards a scientific psychiatric nosology (*Archives of General Psychiatry, 30*:154, 1974); Spitzer, R. L., and Fleiss, J. L.: A re-analysis of the reliability of psychiatric diagnosis (*British Journal of Psychiatry, 125*:341); Zubin, J., Salzinger, K., Fleiss, J. L., Gurland, B., Spitzer, R. L., Endicott, J., and Sutton, S.: Biometric approach to psychopathology (*Annual Review of Psychology, 26*; 621, 1975); Blashfield, R. K. and Draguns, J. G.: Toward a taxonomy of psychopathology: The purpose of psychiatric classification (*British Journal of Psychiatry, 129*:574, 1976). Each of these articles presents a thoughtful consideration of the problems of psychiatric taxonomy. The authors are not wild men simply attacking the establishment. They are serious scholars dedicated to improving the situation.

Inquirer: But at least he has hallucinations?

Young
Psychiatrist: You sound like you are going to question my defini-
                     tion of schizophrenia. I am just going by what I learn-
                     ed in my residency and by what the books say.

Inquirer: But clinicians and books and research literature do *not*
                     agree. Many in the field do not see the problem, or see it
                     as a fundamental problem, or, if they do, they cannot
                     quite characterize what is wrong and what should be
                     done about it. I will try to spell out for you more precise-
                     ly what the crisis involves. For instance, one textbook
                     will say hallucinations characterize schizophrenia and
                     another will say these are neither necessary nor suffi-
                     cient conditions to make a diagnosis of this disorder.
                     Whom do we believe? The simple truth is that the
                     category that we label "schizophrenia" is unreliable.[6]

---

[6]The Inquirer had best step carefully here. He is somewhat recklessly challenging a sacred cow. If there is one disorder of whose existence psychiatrists are certain, it is schizophrenia. The struggles about this major mental illness have had a tortured history over the past century. At first it was call-ed "dementia praecox," which at least had the virtue of suggesting two measurements and providing for prediction to a criterion of poor outcome. Having metrics, the category was refutable. Since 1911, the terms have been replaced by schizophrenia, at least among English-speaking psychiatrists. In some European countries, however, the disorder is still called "dementia praecox."

A diagnosis of schizophrenia predicts to no particular outcome or prognosis, and, hence, its predictive validity as a category is untestable. Precisely what the disorder is, and how it is to be characterized, remains obscure. It lacks construct validity in that there is no interview-independent test yielding a value or measure characteristic only of schizophrenics. Being a conglomeration without a structure, it is not a natural kind, a conceptual class that will be discussed at length in Dialogue V.

Schizophrenia subtypes come and go. Thirty years ago, catatonic schizophrenia was common and paranoid schizophrenia less common. Now their relative frequencies are reversed, and to about the same degree, which offers a hint as to what has happened to psychiatrists' beliefs about the disorder. The once-frequent hebephrenic schizophrenia has all but disappeared from the lexicons of modern psychiatric hospitals.

The Inquirer is not asserting that people who have delusions or hallucinations or bizarre thoughts do not exist. To claim this would be patently absurd. When one questions the reliability of a category, one does not question the existence of *some* individuals who fit the category's definition. The question is, "How many of the class members with the same label fit?" If most do not, then the small remainder constitutes "classic" or "textbook" cases which serve as ideal prototypes, exemplars, with the majority of cases clustered around them at varying distances of approximate resemblance. The crucial scientific question is, How are the standards characterizing the prototype arrived at? By a committee vote? By disciplined empirical inquiry? If one studies what experts *believe* to constitute the defining characteristics of a prototype, one is studying a belief system that may or may not correspond to the structure of reality. The experts' beliefs may be grounded solely in their indoctrination and training experience. See Cantor, N., Smith, E., French, R. deS., and Mezzich, J.: Psychiatric diagnosis as prototype categorization (*Journal of Abnormal Psychology*, *89*:181, 1980).

Young
Psychiatrist: Do you mean to tell me that there is no such thing as schizophrenia? There are now hundreds and thousands of books and articles in the literature on the subject. Billions of dollars have been poured into the treatment of schizophrenia. We have large government institutes and private foundations sponsoring schizophrenia research. Entire journals and periodic bulletins are concerned with it.[7] One or two percent of our population has schizophrenia. Millions of people all over the world have been diagnosed as schizophrenic. Do you mean to tell me the whole field is the victim of a giant delusion? You can't be serious. Is this a variation of the emperor's clothes gag? Or are you one of those radical nuts who just likes to attack the establishment?

Inquirer: But I did not deny the existence of schizophrenia: I said something different. I said it is not a reliable category.

Young
Psychiatrist: Then what do you mean by "reliable category"?[8]

Inquirer: There are at least two sorts of reliability to be considered in this context: (1) interjudge agreements; (2) intrajudge agreements over time. The first is the more fundamental. When several experts observe and assess information about a patient, they should agree on a diagnosis a reasonable percentage of the time given that they have the same information and are using the same classification scheme. If judges agree, that does not necessarily mean they are correct. But if

---

[7] Although it may seem to be the house organ of schizophrenia, the *Schizophrenia Bulletin* open-mindedly publishes research articles and reviews that are severely critical of the concept of schizophrenia. For example, see Fenton, W. S., Mosher, L. R., and Matthews, S. M.: Diagnosis of schizophrenia: A critical review of current diagnostic systems (*Schizophrenia Bulletin*, 1:452, 1981). This article reviews the merits of five diagnostic systems, indicating that none of them is satisfactory, and warning of a premature closure in elevating a single system such as DSM-III to an official status of being the final word that it does not deserve.

[8] The term *reliable* is easily misunderstood because it has so many different meanings. In courts of law, a reliable witness is one who is believed because he is considered to be telling the truth. A reliable car is one that does not break down for long periods of time. Reliable knowledge is that knowledge we would trust in deciding what to believe and how to act.

they cannot agree, at least at above chance level, then something is amiss. Their diagnoses are unreliable in the ordinary sense of not representing knowledge one would rely on in making important decisions.

Young
Psychiatrist: Of course. But surely experts agree on schizophrenia, otherwise we wouldn't have all that literature I mentioned and all that research and 1 percent of the entire population being schizophrenic.

Inquirer: I realize it is hard for you to accept that the huge and impressive systems that have grown up around the chimera of schizophrenia might be illusory or represent a major conceptual mistake. But isn't it possible? There are lots of similar historical examples. During the eighteenth century, the French Academy of Sciences once declared that meteorites simply did not exist, although they seemed massively and incandescently obvious to everybody else.[9] For awhile, some physicists in this century believed in N-rays.[10] It took medicine two centuries to abandon the practice of bleeding patients, often with leeches. Once simple statistics about the successes and failures of bloodletting were collected, the practice gradually became abandoned.[11] It is *not* the case that psychiatrists agree about schizophrenia, as you can discover for yourself in the literature to which I referred you. Would you make a serious decision about a patient when experts cannot agree on the diagnosis at better than chance levels? For example, would you sterilize her?

---

[9] Upon hearing of this orotund pronouncement, many museums threw away their precious meteorites. See Polanyi, M.: *Personal Knowledge: Towards a Post-Critical Philosophy* (Chicago, University of Chicago Press, 1958, p. 138).

[10] The French Academy awarded the reputable French physicist, Blondot, a prize for his discovery of N-rays in 1903. Coming soon after the convincing discovery of X-rays, the mysterious rays turned out to be an illusion or hallucination on the part of the physicist. See Gardner, M.: *Fads and Fallacies in the Name of Science*, 2nd ed. (New York Dover, 1957, p. 345).

[11] But not without a struggle over several generations. See Feinstein, A. R.: *Clincial Judgment* (Baltimore, Williams and Wilkins, 1967, p. 220). The relatively unsung hero who initiated the eventual abandonment was Pierre Ch. A. Louis (1787-1872), who simply counted and compared the results of patients treated in various ways. His treatise appeared in 1836. As we have come to expect from reading history, our hero was vilified and lauded. Incidentally even today, in some quarters, physicians are still called leeches, but perhaps for different reasons.

Young
Psychiatrist: Surely, a rhetorical question.[12] So to be precise, let's say
the term *schizophrenia* does not label a reliable category.
Does that mean there is no such thing as schizophrenia;
that it's a pure myth as, for example, Szasz claims?

Inquirer: Szasz asserts that all mental illness is a myth.[13] But
Szasz thinks of illness in purely biophysical-disease
terms. His vantage point is highly physical and body-
bound, ignoring the effects of the socio-symbolic environment. His model of an illness is paresis, an infectious disease in which physical damage to cells and
tissue can be demonstrated. He does not take into account that there can be a scientific concept of a
disorder in which there is nothing physically "wrong."
For example, in a computer system, the hardware ar-
chitecture can be physically intact while there is an error in the symbolic program producing undesirable
pathological behavior.[14]

Young
Psychiatrist: I don't want to get into computer talk first; because I
don't understand the contraption in the first place
and, second, I don't think people are computers.[15]
Let's stick to the problem of diagnosis, which I think I

---

[12]He means "no!" What he overlooks is that only 30 years ago over 40,000 hospitalized
men and women in the United States who received a diagnosis of schizophrenia were steril-
ized in the heriditarian belief that it would reduce the frequency of this disorder in the population. See Gamble, C. J.: The sterilization of psychotic patients under state law (*American
Journal of Psychiatry, 105*: 60, 1948). It is a tribute to the resiliency of people deemed
schizophrenic that they have survived bowel resections, teeth removal, metrazol shock, insulin shock, electric shock, starvation, brain surgery and the currently fashionable ad-
ministration of drugs having formidable short-range and long-range side effects, both
physically and socially.

[13]See Szasz, T. S.: *The Myth of Mental Illness* (New York, Harper and Row, 1961). Szasz, an
experienced psychiatrist, is an extensively published critic of just about everything that is
happening in psychiatry.

[14]All of a sudden, the Inquirer unloads a benumbing computer analogy into the argument. If
the Young Psychiatrist were familiar with the concepts and vocabulary involved, this would
be a legitimate move. But since he is not, the comparison is premature and even a bit unfair.
Other sorts of experts should have a chance at this loaded computer perspective. And they
will in the Dialogues to come.

[15]The Young Psychiatrist, being no beginner in psychiatric argumentation, snaps back with a
point of his own. Nothing has been said about people being computers. But there will be in
Dialogue VI with "The Mind Scientist."

know at least something about from four years of medical school, a year's internship in medicine and three years of psychiatric residency. When you say psychiatry is weak at its foundations, you can't mean that all diagnostic categories in psychiatry are as unreliable as schizophrenia?[16]

Inquirer: Not necessarily. Reliability generally depends on the variables involved and level of description being used. Paranoia, in the sense of having persecutory delusions, is highly reliable with 90-100% agreements.[17] But the diagnosis is not difficult in extreme cases. People can often identify it among their relatives and acquaintances. The closer one stands

---

[16]Perhaps the Young Psychiatrist gives up on schizophrenia too easily. He could point to a large body of self-described "hard-science" work claiming a genetic factor in schizophrenia. He might even quote Kety's joke, "If schizophrenia is a myth, it is a myth with a large genetic component." He would, in turn, be shot down by the contradictory nature of the evidence. For example, among the Feighner criteria for schizophrenia is a family history of schizophrenia. (Let us charitably ignore the potential circularities here.) One study, however, showed that among eighty-nine patients receiving a diagnosis of schizophrenia, eleven satisfied the Feighner criteria (except for family history) but none of the nineteen first-degree relatives could be found to have schizophrenia. See Taylor, M. A. and Abrams, R.: A critique of the St. Louis psychiatric research criteria for schizophrenia (*American Journal of Psychiatry, 132*: 1276, 1975).

Another study of 580 patients showed a low morbidity risk for schizophrenia (2.11%) among first-degree relatives of patients diagnosed under the Feighner system but a *higher* morbidity risk for affective disease (5.5%) among the relatives! See Winokur, G., Morrison, J., Clancy, J., and Crowe, R.: The Iowa 500: II. A blind family history comparison of mania, depression, and schizophrenia (*Archives of General Psychiatry, 27*:462, 1972). In a blind study of 199 first-degree relatives of 39 cases of schizophrenia, *no* cases of even "possible" schizophrenia were found. See Pope, H. J., Jonas, J. M., Cohen, B. M., and Lapinski, J. F.: Failure to find evidence of schizophrenia in first-degree relatives of schizophrenic probands (*American Journal of Psychiatry, 139*:826, 1982). Geneticists themselves find research work in the field next to impossible because the patients called schizophrenic form too heterogeneous a group for effective investigation. See Penrose, L. S.: A critical survey of schizophrenia genetics (*Modern Perspectives in World Psychiatry, 2*:3, 1971). Penrose compares the vague class "schizophrenia" to the vague class "epilepsy" and despairs of finding anything so precise as a genetic factor in such ill-defined categories.

Family studies, twin studies, and adoption studies have been too imprecise to answer the genetic question in the absence of a genetic marker. Down's syndrome, by contrast, is much better defined and has a genetic marker. If one uses one discipline (the primary) to investigate the problems of another (the secondary), no matter how precise the primary is, it can't get very far when the secondary's categories or kinds are so vaguely defined that they cannot be agreed upon.

[17]See Spitzer, R. L., Forman, Y. B. W., and Nee, J.: DSM-III field trials: I. Initial interrater diagnostic reliability (*American Journal of Psychiatry, 136*:815, 1979) Also, cf. Hilf, F.: Dynamic content analysis (*Archives of General Psychiatry, 32*:97, 1975).

to direct observational terms, the greater the agreement. You and I would easily agree that a patient is crying. We might even agree that he is depressed. But whether it is neurotic depression, a psychotic depression, unipolar or bipolar, then disagreement mounts. The more abstract the category, the less reliable it becomes for us.

Young
Psychiatrist: Isn't the category called "organic brain disease" a reliable one?

Inquirer: Yes, the agreements here are quite good, ranging above an 80 percent level, although a great deal depends on the particular organic brain disease involved.[18] Strokes and brain tumors are easy to diagnose, but senile dementia can be readily confused with depression.[19] When we have some objective signs, as we do in cases of strokes and brain tumors, our judgments are more reliable.

Young
Psychiatrist: But we use signs as well as symptoms in psychiatry as indicators of disorder.

Inquirer: Not as many signs as symptoms. A diagnostic sign in medicine is what can be observed. For example, yellow skin color can be a sign of liver disease.[20] A symptom is what the patient experiences, complains of, and reports on, for example, feeling sad. Notice

---

[18]Cf. Spitzer, DSM-III field trials. It may seem paradoxical that one of the most reliable categories in psychiatry is a neurological one. But nature is not always divided up the way medical specialties are. Patients with organic brain diseases who present behavior problems are taken care of by psychiatrists, not neurologists. Senile dementia is an example in point.
[19]See Wells, C. E.: Pseudodementia (*American Journal of Psychiatry*, 136:895, 1979).
[20]Semiotic, the science of signs, originated with the Stoic Greek medical tradition that interpreted diagnosis and treatment as sign processes. Cf. Morris, C.: *Signs, Language and Behavior* (New York, Braziller, 1955, p. 285), as well as Morris, C.: *Signification and Significance*, (Cambridge, MIT Press, 1964, p. 1). Charles Sanders Peirce (1839-1914), an outsized American thinker, offered a triadic definition of a sign as something which stands to somebody for something in some respect or capacity. For Peirce, "all this universe is perfused with signs, if it is not composed exclusively of signs." Cf. Peirce, C. S.: In Hartshorne, C. and Weiss, P. (Eds.): *Collected Papers* (Cambridge, Harvard University Press, 1931-1976). These dialogues will become perfused with talk of signs as well as with Peirce, the Thinker's Thinker. One of us (KMC) read him for years without hearing his name pronounced. Hence, he did not initially grasp whom a professor was referring to when he mentioned "purse."

we do not *see* or *hear* or examine a disorder; we *infer* its presence from what can be seen or heard or examined. Most of the indicators we use in psychiatric diagnosis consist of the patients' complaints of "troubles" and symptoms. Here, again, we have difficulties. The patient says he is sad, but is he "really" sad? A clinician might claim that a patient is not sad, but angry. Judges have been shown to agree at only the 46 percent level on just the presence or absence of symptoms.[21]

Young
Psychiatrist: This is getting terrible. You are shredding up what I have been taught in psychiatry. Maybe it is you and the authorities you quote who are as wrong as the French Academy of Sciences was. Oliver Cromwell once pleaded, "I beseech you in the bowels of Christ, think it possible you may be mistaken." How am I going to get out in the real world of making a living by practicing psychiatry if the diagnostic system cannot be relied on? If we don't know what we are talking about, as you claimed initially, how are we going to know what we are doing?

Inquirer: Exactly. But don't despair. As a practitioner in that "real" world, you will soon learn that experienced clinicians do not use the official diagnostic system much, either in helping their patients or in informally communicating with one another. They rely on their own assessment of facts about the patient. They have their own personal "diagnoses" or evaluation of an individual patient who might be at various "distances" from the learned textbook case, the prototype they were indoctrinated with. Practitioners treat *clinical phenomena* more than diseases.

Medical reasoning is concerned more with making decisions and deciding what to do next, than it is with *the* diagnosis. In your medical internship when a

---

[21]See Kreitman, N., Sainsbury, F., Morrisey, J., Towers, J., and Scrivener, J.: The reliability of psychiatric assessment: an analysis (*Journal of Mental Science, 107*:887, 1961). What do we see and what do we hear when we examine a patient? What we need here is a philosopher to help us with these elementary concepts. One will shortly appear in Dialogue IV with "The Metaphysician."

patient suffered a myocardial infarction, you gave
him morphine for pain, vasopressor for shock, and
put him in bed. You were not treating the infarct; you
were treating its attendant phenomena. If you ask
an experienced psychiatrist for the diagnosis of a patient he has been treating for several months, he will
have to stop and think up an official diagnosis if he
thinks that is what you want from him by your question.[22] His main concern *now* may be with the fact
that the patient does not have a job.[23] In treatment, a
clinician uses his fact space, not the official diagnosis
space.

To go back to my example of referral of a schizophrenic patient in actual clinical practice, I would *not*
refer you a case of schizophrenia unless we shared the
same code terms for the disorder.[24] I would describe

---

[22]Psychiatrists, of all people, should be experts on the dialectic of questions and answers. Who
is asking what of whom? Besides the content of a question, what is the intention of the ques-
tioner? What sort of answer would satisfy him to terminate the questioning? It is now a standard joke that a psychiatrist tends to answer a question by asking a question (e.g. the classical
response, "Why do you ask?")

[23]A psychiatric patient usually presents a multiplicity of problems and troubled states.
Patient-states are variable over time. Hence, probability theory and its accompanying
statistics are appropriate for the analysis of patient variability. This point was recognized
quite awhile ago by the mathematician Von Mises: "The entire field of phenomena, like
dream images, slips, et cetera, seems much more similar to the type of physical events with
which the calculus of probability is concerned than to the type of physical events which led to
the concept of causality." Cf. Von Mises, R.: *Positivism: A Study in Human Understanding* (Cambridge,
Harvard University Press, 1951, p. 238). (A translation of Von Mises' Kleines Lehrbuch des
Positivismus, 1939.) For a thorough treatment of the implications of a probabilistic or stochastic
viewpoint, see Chassan, J. B.: *Research Design in Clinical Psychology and Psychiatry*, 2nd Ed. (New
York, Appleton-Century-Crofts, 1979), as well as Chassan, J. B.: Stochastic models of the single
case as the basis of clinical research design (*Behavioral Science*, 6:42, 1961).

[24]When people familiar with one another communicate, their signs often consist of shared abbreviations for much longer descriptions of complex concepts. Such code terms can provide a
spurious basis for "independent" judgment agreements. The Inquirer defined his use of the
term *reliability* to mean interjudge agreement. It is not only agreement that is important, but
how the agreement is arrived at. Judges must agree independently. If two supposedly independent psychiatric judges share the code term *loose associations* to signify schizophrenia and
only schizophrenia, then the simple mention of "loose associations" by one judge gives away
the diagnosis he is considering to the other judge. Thus, diagnostic judges of patient data, to
be independent, should not be in the same room nor be able to send *any* signal to one another.
The quantum-theoretical term for this is "Einstein separability," referring to the fact that a
physical system cannot influence another physical system outside of its light cone. See
d'Espagnat, B.: The quantum theory and reality (*Scientific American, 241*:158, 1979).

to you a twenty-year-old college student who can't concentrate, has insomnia and loss of appetite, who fears he is going crazy and wants help. I would ask you if you have time to see him. This is the way it is done in actual clinical practice. It is when you have to write down a diagnosis for a third-party payment for a National Health Insurance Plan that you will have some trouble.

Young
Psychiatrist: Isn't this what DSM-III is supposed to help me with?
Inquirer: It is supposed to but it will and it won't. The book DSM-III represents the psychiatric profession's heroic response to the inadequacy of its earlier efforts, such as DSM-II, to provide a "useful" classification of the disorders that patients present. In preparing DSM-III, committees of experts reviewed all of the relevant literature to decide on what characteristics patients actually demonstrated and how these characteristics clustered together. With new data on the natural history (i.e. long-term course), response to somatic treatments (e.g. drugs, ECT), physiologic concomitants, associated family histories, and associated physical abnormalities of certain "symptom clusters," it seemed possible to create new categories that would be more logically consistent, i.e. that would be descriptive, and would not make confusing allusions to etiology, except where etiology is fairly well known. The categories would have more precise definitions, and could be operationalized in terms of prototypes.[25]

Young
Psychiatrist: Operationalized? What does that mean?
Inquirer: It means each category is not only defined, but a set of criteria is specified such that if a patient had a large number of them, he would be an exemplar or prototype of the class. This allows a clinician to determine which patients are instances of the category under considera-

---

[25]American Psychiatric Association. DSM-III, 1980, p. 7.

tion by comparing them to the exemplar.[26]

Young
Psychiatrist: That sounds ideal. Does it succeed?

Inquirer: Not adequately, I'm afraid. First, the interrater reliability of its categories leaves much to be desired. Using the authors' own criterion of a kappa agreement at the 0.7 level (i.e. the level of agreement is corrected for agreeing by chance alone),[27] 47 percent of the major categories of adult disorders were, after field testing, found to be unreliable even in the hands of clinicians who were interested enough in DSM-III to respond to advertisements and participate in the field trials.[28] In similarly committed hands, only one of eleven of the major categories of disorders of childhood or adolescence reached the 0.7 level of reliability in the last field trial. By the way, that one reliable category is based on the fact that two clinicians agreed that *one* child had an anxiety disorder! We are not told, however, if they agreed upon which of the three subcategories of anxiety disorder the child had.[29]

I should add that the field trials were conducted with less than rigorous methodology. In one-third of the cases, two clinicians' category assignments were made after simultaneous interview of a patient, during which there may well have been considerable information exchanged between the clinicians about each other's thinking; for example, by which ques-

---

[26]A definition states the meaning of a concept; a criterion is a test that provides evidence for the concept. We define monozygotic twins as stemming from a single zygote. Given, say, two adults, what tests could we subject them to in order to establish that they are monozygotic twins? Such tests would serve as evidential criteria for the concept, but not the definition of the concept. Pure operationists confuse tests with meaning.

[27]When two judges agree, their chance agreement is a function of how many cases in the sample they agree to call well or ill. Kappa is statistic of intraclass correlations that corrects for chance agreement between two, and only two, judges.

[28]American Psychiatric Association. DSM-III, 1980, p. 470.

[29]American Psychiatric Association. DSM-III, 1980, p. 471. The example illustrates that one must look carefully at the data before evaluating easily read abstracts or conclusions at the end of a paper. Sweeping conclusions have been made about the genetic factor in schizophrenia based on relatives of only six cases of chronic schizophrenia diagnosed by DSM-II criteria. See Kety, S.S., Rosenthal, D., and Wender, P.H.: Genetic relationships within the schizophrenic spectrum: evidence from adoption studies. In Spitzer, R.L. and Klein, D.F. (Eds.): *Current Issues in Psychiatric Diagnosis* (New York, Raven Press, p. 213).

tions were asked, how they were answered, how and where much emphasis was placed, detail pursued, etc. In the other two-thirds of the cases, the clinicians were encouraged to exchange data about the cases when one had "relevant data" that the other didn't. One wonders how much the reliability coefficient of the category "schizophrenic disorder" (which reached 0.81) owes to one clinician reporting to another that "the patient reported an auditory hallucination in which a voice keeps up a running commentary on his thoughts, and he said that he's never told anyone about it before."[30] The category schizophrenic disorder is the only one in which that particular symptom is described, so such a communication might well lead to diagnostic agreement that would not be representative of the "real life" reliability of the category.

Also, DSM-III has, I presume in the interest of increasing "coverage" (i.e. reducing the number of persons whose disorder cannot be classified), adopted the use of "atypical" subcategories for most of the major categories of disorder. For example, "atypical anxiety disorder" is defined as "the individual appears to have an anxiety disorder that does not meet the criteria for any of the above specified conditions." Unfortunately, no criteria are given for deciding which patients, "appear to have an anxiety disorder." This category reminds me of a classification described to me by a biologist friend of mine. It includes categories like "those that are included in this classification," but most resembles DSM-III in its category — "others." Unlike DSM-III, though, it wasn't created by a committee of experts, and it's not meant to be taken seriously.[31]

---

[30]In some studies, inflated kappas are achieved by collapsing the judgments "illness probable" and "illness definite" into an agreement of "illness present." See Spitzer, R. L., Endicott, J., and Robins, E.: Clinical criteria for psychiatric diagnosis and DSM-III (*American Journal of Psychiatry, 132*:1187, 1975).

[31]This possibly apocryphal classification scheme will be outlined in the dialogue to come with "The Biological Scientist," Dialogue V.

In a less critical vein, however, I must acknowledge that DSM-III is aware of most of its weaknesses. Regarding the classification of personality disorders, it observes that a high order of inference is required to "see" the essential features of personality disorder and later admits that "the kappas for the specific personality disorder are quite low and range from 0.26 to 0.75." Moreover, in an attempt to add characteristics (instead of using just signs, symptoms and course), DSM-III has gone to a multi-axial system whereby simultaneous assessment along several different axes can be made.[32] Thus, a major psychiatric diagnosis, a personality diagnosis, diagnoses of physical illness(es), the level of psychosocial stress and highest level of adaptive functioning in the past year all can be specified for each patient.

In this way, DSM-III might stimulate the collection of data that may, in the future, lead to improvement of the scheme. But don't get too excited, because the use of the last three axes is described as "optional" which in the real world translates to "nobody will do it."

This leads us to the heart of the matter, the real insurmountable obstacle that DSM-III fails to overcome, and that is, its own goals. Pages 2 and 3 list no less than 10 goals of DSM-III, including "Maintaining acceptability to clinicians and researchers of varying theoretical orientation" and "avoiding the introduction of terminology and concepts that break with tradition, except when clearly needed."[33] Following the list of goals, DSM-III goes on to assure that each goal has been afforded equal weight and that the overall document is designed to attain the least possible amount of "overall goal-achievement failure." The sad truth is that a truly scientific effort may have produced a scientifically reasonable

---

[32]American Psychiatric Association. DSM-III, 1980.
[33]American Psychiatric Association. DSM-III, 1980, p. 2.

diagnostic scheme; instead, we have a politically motivated compromise between differing interpretations of the data, outright dogma, and propaganda.

Young
Psychiatrist: You have your points but you miss my point. I am going to have to use DSM-III!

Inquirer: And you will use it, judiciously, I'm sure, if you want to make a living. You will fill out forms in order to get paid by third-party carriers. For remuneration, you will, in part, make-believe just like all of us do. It is not your job as a practitioner to overhaul the classification scheme or to construct a new one. That is the job of psychiatric scientists and investigators.[34]

Young
Psychiatrist: Enough already. I'm going to have to talk to someone else about all this. Something is wrong someplace.[35]

Inquirer: Without doubt. Why don't you talk to the Old Psychiatrist?[36]

---

[34]Practitioners in the community are able to take care of patients with their current state of knowledge. They are not in a position to construct new classifications or devise new therapies. It is the function of universities to constructively criticize current practices and to responsibly test out improvements on them. Testing a new drug, for example, requires scientific and statistical resources available in a university but not available in a practitioner's office. He can *use* the results, but he cannot generate them systematically.

[35]When shared perspectives, paradigms, models, or sets of beliefs of a discipline are shown by repeated experience to be unreliable, a crisis develops and the field or specialty becomes ripe for fundamental change. For a thorough discussion of historical examples, see Kuhn, T.: *The Structure of Scientific Revolutions*, 2nd Ed. (Chicago, University of Chicago Press, 1970). A field plagued with failures does not give up its current paradigm, however, unless an alternative is available. In the crisis of a storm, a ship with a broken rudder is better than no ship at all.

[36]The Inquirer realizes that his critical position is not easily acceptable to the Young Psychiatrist. Hence he refers him to the Old Psychiatrist who provides a much better role-model for a practitioner and who may be more reassuring about the uncertainties and anxieties of entering the difficult field of actually practicing psychiatry.

THE OLD PSYCHIATRIST

AFTER medical school, the Old Psychiatrist interned in medicine and practiced medicine for a few years before entering a four-year psychiatric residency at a leading university hospital. He underwent psychoanalysis and now practices psychiatry in a nearby community. He is on the clinical faculty of a university hospital, supervises residents in psychiatry, consults with community mental health workers, and specializes in the current fashions, one of which is psychopharmacology. He is taken as a model (Dr. Compleat) by many young psychiatrists. He has white hair and wears a long white coat.

Old
Psychiatrist: I have just talked with the Young Psychiatrist. What is all this crapola you have been giving him about the classification scheme? Are you trying to give him an illusionectomy?

Inquirer: I told him the classification scheme was mainly unreliable. I know it, you know it and a lot of people know it.[1] You and I are both afraid to insist on it too loudly because we don't want to foul the nest. Also, we don't want to be appointed to serve on a committee

---

[1]See Koestler, A.: Can Psychiatrists Be Trusted? In *The Heel of Achilles, Essays 1968-1973* (New York, Random House, 1974). Koestler cites the cross-national studies indicating that if he were admitted to a psychiatric hospital in England, he would have a ten-times higher chance of being classified as manic-depressive than if he were admitted to a psychiatric hospital in the United States, where he would have a 33 percent higher chance of being classified as schizophrenic. See Cooper, J. E., Kendell, R. E., Gurland, B. J., et al.: Cross-national study of diagnosis of mental disorders (*American Journal of Psychiatry, 125*:21, 1969) and Kendell, R. E., Cooper, J. E., Gourlay, A. J., Copeland, J. R.M., Sharpe, L., and Gurland, B. J. Diagnostic criteria of American and British psychiatrists (*Archives of General Psychiatry, 25*:123, 1971). There have been several attempts to understand the sources of disagreement. See Kendell, R. E.: *The Role of Diagnosis in Psychiatry* (Oxford, Blackwell, 1975, p. 70). In one study of a filmed interview, one-third of the American psychiatrists classified the patient as schizophrenic, but *not a single* British psychiatrist offered that diagnosis of the same patient. Gleeful critics have a field day with such data. But it should be noted that the disagreements were discovered by research on the part of psychiatrists themselves who are seeking to understand and correct the situation.

to rectify it. Anything is possible until it goes to a committee.

Old
Psychiatrist: The Young Psychiatrist is a bit upset. He has to practice, to take action, in order to make a living. To act, one must believe the action is justified. If you tell him he doesn't know what he's doing or even what he's talking about, and he believes it, he cannot act. He cannot sit around and just talk about these things like you academic pedants. He has to *do* something for his patients.[2]

Inquirer: In the long run it should help a field, if not an individual, to face and know the truth. An accurate specification of ignorance can be helpful. I told the Young Psychiatrist he can still practice. He simply doesn't need the official classification scheme to help his patients with currently available techniques.

Old
Psychiatrist: Why not?

Inquirer: Because he is treating them and their troubles and not their diagnoses. By the way, did you use DSM-II?

Old
Psychiatrist: No. I mislaid my copy. DSM-II did not make much sense to me to begin with. It listed definitions of syndromes, but most all of the syndromes had the same symptoms. Also, there was no way of knowing how to apply criteria to a particular case in order to identify the patient as having a particular disorder. I gave up on it. To be diagnosed schizophrenic, did the patient have to have delusions *and* hallucinations *and* loose thought associations *and* flat affect *and* be withdrawn? Or just two of these? How about one? Manic patients

---

[2]Again, as in note 1, Dialogue I, we witness the pressure on the practitioner as technologist to act and to act successfully in getting things done efficiently. To accomplish this, he needs rules that prescribe how to proceed in order to achieve a goal. As practitioner, the psychiatrist works under constraints of urgency, compassion, cost, and effectiveness. He cannot wait as a scientist can. For a wide-ranging discussion of the philosophy of technology, see Bunge, M.: The philosophical richness of technology. In Suppe, F., and Asquith, P. D. (Eds.): *Proceedings of the 1976 Biennial Meeting of the Philosophy of Science Association*, Vol. II (East Lansing, Philosophy of Science Association, 1977, p. 153).

can have hallucinations. Well, maybe then they are not manic but schizophrenic, or maybe they are both, or maybe there is something we can call *schizo-affective* disorder.

Inquirer: So you agree with me about difficulties in using DSM-II?

Old
Psychiatrist: Why do you fulminate so against these manuals? Everybody knows they are the outcome of professional compromises typical of committees. Their main use is administrative and remunerative. And why do you keep picking on DSM-II? It may be better in some respects than DSM-III. In a recent study of childhood and adolescent psychiatric disorders, the average rater agreement using DSM-III with the expected diagnosis of the authors was less than 50 percent.[3] I guess I can agree with you about the doubtful value of DSM manuals, but not about the position you took with the Young Psychiatrist about diagnosis.

Inquirer: Where did I go wrong in my argument with him?[4]

Old
Psychiatrist: In practice, you have to have some sort of evaluation to start with. That is, you need at least some concept of disorder, an idea about what is wrong with the patient.

Inquirer: Laing claims there is nothing wrong with the patient but that there is something wrong with society.[5]

Old
Psychiatrist: Why couldn't there be something wrong with both the patient and society? Let's face clinical reality. If a

---

[3]See Cantwell, D. P., Russell, A. T., Mattison, R., and Will, L.: A comparison of DSM-II and DSM-III in the diagnosis of childhood psychiatric disorders. I. Agreement with expected diagnosis. II. Interrater agreement (*Archives of General Psychiatry, 36*:1208 and 1217, 1979). Somewhat ironically, the senior author served on the committee that formulated DSM-III.
[4]We cannot believe the Inquirer is serious in this confession. Perhaps he senses an ally for his position and tries to draw out arguments he may not have heard before. These arguments, or their counters, may come in handy later as ammunition in dialogues with other disputants.
[5]Cf. Laing, R. D.: *The Politics of Experience* (New York, Pantheon, 1967). Laing can be viewed as the British gadfly counterpart of the American Szasz, although the latter does not agree that schizophrenia is a superior form of adjustment.

middle-aged woman is running nude down the streets of a city, shouting and swearing at people, smearing her feces on herself and passersby, sobbing face down in the gutter when the police arrive — something is wrong. The police take her in and try to find out who she is so as to contact her family. They call a doctor. They know there is something wrong and that this type of wrongness is not criminal. Notice Laing doesn't deny, as I take it you do, that there is such a thing as schizophrenia. He believes schizophrenia is a creative adaptation to a sick society.

Inquirer: I don't deny the existence of schizophrenia as a conceptual category. What I assert is that the concept is so vague and ill-defined that calling a patient schizophrenic helps neither us nor him. In fact, such a documented diagnosis can have pernicious consequences when the patient tries to get a job or enter medical school. Individuals now placed in the class represent a very heterogenous group like the class "everyone within three miles of this building." Such a group would possess such a wildly disjunctive set of properties as to be useless as a concept for both treatment and research purposes.[6] Lower level, ordinary language descriptions are perhaps more reliable, but you pay a price for them; they can't readily be generalized. It's an old joke that the only reliable diagnosis in psychiatry is the patient's name. Just to describe the patient is to use a classification of sorts because the words of English themselves designate concepts.

Old Psychiatrist: You can describe someone as depressed without saying he has a DEPRESSION in the official-scheme sense.

Inquirer: You are saying the patient can be depressed without having the disorder depression?

---

[6]This is a bit hasty. What if you were studying the effects of radiation leakage from a nuclear reactor housed in the building? This group would be a proper entity for study. The Old Psychiatrist will make this point later regarding the goals of a classification.

Old
Psychiatrist: Why not? The trouble with saying he has the disorder
                 depression is that someone else will say, "No — he has
                 the disorder anxiety neurosis with depressive
                 features," and I will say "No — he has the disorder
                 depression with anxiety features as secondary" and
                 away we go to Disneyland. I have been through this
                 muddle hundreds of times in psychiatric case con-
                 ferences.

Inquirer: Why not weight the symptoms? If depression is
                 greater than anxiety, call it a depression.

Old
Psychiatrist: Who does the weighting, using what method of as-
                 signment? And how are the weights to be inter-
                 preted? It has been reported that if British
                 psychiatrists observe "affect" in the patient, they call
                 him manic-depressive, whereas American psychia-
                 trists, given the same patient, call him schizophren-
                 ic.[7]

Inquirer: That must not be very reassuring to you.

Old
Psychiatrist: There are worse examples. But I will defend
                 psychiatry on the grounds that the same thing goes on
                 in medicine, and medicine is supposed to have a
                 reliable diagnostic system.

Inquirer: Surely it is more reliable than ours.

Old
Psychiatrist: It depends on whether laboratory findings or other
                 objective measures are included in the facts of the
                 case.[8] And what are thought of as objective measures
                 may not be all that objective.[9] Experienced radiolo-

---

[7]This is the startling discrepancy footnoted in this dialogue (see note 1).

[8]The status of "objective" findings in medicine is reviewed in Galen, R. S., and Gambino, S.
R.: *Beyond Normality: The Predictive Value and Efficiency of Medical Diagnosis* (New York, John
Wiley, 1975), and also in DeDombal, F. T.: How "objective" is medical data? In DeDombal,
F. T., and Grenay, F. (Eds.): *Decision Making and Medical Care: Can Information Science Help?*
(Amsterdam, North Holland, 1976). The problem of observer variation plagues every field
from quantum physics to medicine and psychiatry.

[9]Observer variability and agreement in a large set of medical tests are discussed in two articles
by Koran, L. M.; The reliability of clinical methods, data, and judgements (*New England
Journal of Medicine, 293*:642 and 695, 1975).

gists reading chest films disagree 30 percent of the time.[10] Over 30 percent of appendectomies are performed on normal appendices.[11]

Hence, there can be great observer variation in even the most sophisticated of medical diagnostic procedures. When I interned in medicine, I heard four specialists agree that a patient had cancer of the stomach, but on operation, only a peptic ulcer was found.

Inquirer: By the way, this illustrates the difference between reliability and validity. The judges agreed, but that didn't imply they were accurate.

Old
Psychiatrist: Obviously. Medicine began to make major progress only in this century when doctors had more than signs and symptoms to go on. The final arbiter became a pathologist. He can just look at the tissue and determine the diagnosis.

Inquirer: It's not always that easy. Take your cancer case. Looking at the same slides of cells, three pathologists will say they are cancerous and three will say they are not.[12] There is still an element of inference-dependent interpretation in what experts see.

Old
Psychiatrist: Granted, but across the board medicine does better than psychiatry.

Inquirer: That may be because the diagnostic process in medicine is better understood. They have lots of variegated evidence to rely on, and they now have computerized mathematical aids in selecting the final diagnosis.

Old
Psychiatrist: That may be so, but I understand there exists in medicine considerable controversy over mathematical

[10]See Herman, P. G., and Hessel, S. J.: Accuracy and its relationship to experience in the interpretaton of chest radiographs (*Investigative Radiology, 10*:62-67, 1975).

[11]See Thomas, E. J., and Mudler, B.: Appendectomy: diagnostic criteria and hospital performance (*Hospital Practice, 4*:72, 1969).

[12]See MacMahon, B., Morrison, A. S., and Ackerman, L. V.: Histological characteristics of breast cancer in Boston and Tokyo (*International Journal of Cancer, 11*:338, 1973).

approaches. You will have to discuss it with someone more scientifically inclined than I am.[13]

Inquirer: Do you think psychiatry should utilize the medical model?

Old
Psychiatrist: Which medical model and whose medical model? I endorse the physiological model in medicine which says that there are certain functions which have a range of values considered normal. Values outside that range are abnormal and represent a disorder. The treatment task is to restore the abnormal values to their normal ranges.

Inquirer: Can you give me a clear example?

Old
Psychiatrist: There is a liver function test in which the normal values range from 0.6 to 1.4. A value below 0.6 indicates the liver is not functioning properly and therefore something must be done to improve liver function.[14]

Inquirer: How did they find out what the normal values were?

Old
Psychiatrist: I don't know how it was done, but I suppose some sort of "normal" or non-sick population was studied. The term *normal* has several meanings in medicine. Sometimes it means a statistical average, sometimes it means what is most commonly encountered, sometimes it means what is best or optimal, and sometimes it means harmless in that nothing has to be done.[15] The

---

[13]The Inquirer is alluding to a large body of work over the past twenty years in computer-aided medical diagnosis (cf. Jacquez, J. A. (Ed.): *Computer Diagnosis and Diagnostic Medicine* (Springfield, Thomas, 1964)). In an attempt to improve diagnostic performance, decision trees, flow charts, and Bayes' theorem have been brought to bear on medical diagnostic problems. See Feinstein, A. R.: An analysis of diagnostic reasoning (*Yale Journal of Biology and Medicine, 46*:212 and 264, 1973). This is not the time to enter into details. The topic will come up again in Dialogue VIII with "The Psychiatric Scientist."

[14]The test and its implications about "normality" are discussed in Murphy, E. A.: The normal and the perils of the sylleptic argument (*Perspectives in Biology and Medicine, 15*:566, 1972).

[15]The many meanings of normal in medicine are also taken up in Murphy, E. A.: *The Logic of Medicine* (Baltimore, Johns Hopkins University Press, 1976, p. 117).

academic clinician likes to ramble on about normality. So maybe you can check with him later.

Inquirer: The question of normal values is crucial for mental disorders. It would be nice if we had something like medicine's physiological model in psychiatry. It would help if we had a set of mental functions, values for their ranges, and a way of measuring or judging whether an individual had values beyond these ranges. But psychology has not provided us with a taxonomy of human mental functions. And perhaps one can't be provided. Notice that in this view of normality there is no need for a concept of disease in the conventional sense.

Old
Psychiatrist: One trouble with the disease concept is that a medically ill patient usually presents several conditions at the same time. A patient can have 10 to 12 "diseases" all interlocking and interacting. It becomes difficult to sort out what is causing what. If there exist 5,000 or even 10,000 diseases, the number of possible combinations is staggering. The question of treating *a* disease then becomes rather useless unless one knows a specific cause of a specific disease and has a high-precision way of countering it, like using antibiotics to treat pneumonia. By the way, another reason I never used DSM-II was because it didn't allow the patient to have multiple disorders. You were either psychotic or neurotic, but not both. In medicine a patient can, and usually does, have more than one disorder.

Inquirer: As a psychiatrist you rely heavily on your medical background in the way you view patients and you treat patients' symptoms with drugs. You probably believe that psychiatric disorders are mainly biological or biochemical in nature.[16]

Old
Psychiatrist: Yes, I believe the ultimate solutions to problems of mental disorder will be at a biochemical level.

---

[16]The Inquirer is blatantly leading on the Old Psychiatrist, but this wise old bird will soon bring him up short, having more to say than the Inquirer originally bargained for.

Inquirer: Perhaps so, but you will be faced with the founda-
             tional problem of a descriptive classification or tax-
             onomy of what is wrong. And you will have to have
             personal or group norms to judge what is abnormal.

Old
Psychiatrist: I agree that a concept of normality is necessary as is a
             concept of disorder, but a classification system isn't.
             The first two don't imply the third at all, and, in fact,
             a great deal of effective medicine is practiced based
             upon norms but not categories. Consider the average
             mother treating her child's fever with aspirin or her
             own headache with codeine. By the way, in the latter
             case there are no "objective signs" at all, but treatment
             is still effective.

Inquirer: But treatment of this sort is hardly representative of
             "medical science" in its most fully developed form.

Old
Psychiatrist: Also agreed. Moreover, I agree with most of your
             premises, but feel you are a bit shrill in your conclu-
             sions. Medicine is a craft, one whose explicit aims are
             the restoration of comfort and function and the pro-
             longation of life. To achieve these aims, medicine has
             of late leaned heavily on a body of knowledge
             generated by basic scientists and refined by clincial
             scientists. But medical practice also relies on cultural
             tradition, custom, shared expectations, magic,
             religion, rhetoric, and good old-fashioned common
             sense.
                 The problem of taxonomy is a vexing problem for
             scientists to be sure, but its solution may or may not
             improve the batting average of the practitioner, whose
             task it is to choose, from all the true statements that
             can be made, which ones are relevant to his goals. If
             you have a ferry boat with limited capacity and your
             task is to get things across a river, it may be entirely
             appropriate to classify things by weight, ignoring
             every other feature. Nobody would claim this to be a
             scientific classification.

Inquirer: Sure it is for its purposes and, although limited, it is based on objective observations.

Old
Psychiatrist: Let me give you a more dramatic example of good "empirical" medicine. A patient that I cared for when I was an intern complained of shaking chills, weakness, shortness of breath, and fever. I ordered blood cultures; the first four grew nothing.[17] His condition worsened, and I became worried! Finally, the fifth blood culture grew *Pseudomonas* (a very virulent bacteria) and I treated him with the appropriate antibiotics and probably saved his life. I daresay the process of determining a diagnosis in this case left a lot to be desired, being based on three "subjective symptoms" and one "objective sign" with a less than 20 percent chance of repeating its own findings. Yet, the patient is alive and well.

Inquirer: But what if the fifth blood culture had also been negative?

Old
Psychiatrist: Then I would have treated him the same way and gotten the same results! How about that for unscientific, but successful medicine? A lot of people are alive today because some emergency room physician was unscientific enough to push a narcotic antagonist (to reverse narcotic overdose) and 50 percent dextrose solution (to reverse insulin-caused hypoglycemia) into their veins while they were still unconscious and could give no history. These ex-patients might be sympathetic to the "pragmatic" modus operandi of the astute clinician.

Inquirer: So we should abandon the aim of a reliable taxonomy and willy-nilly treat patients using everything in our black bags?

Old
Psychiatrist: Please. What I propose is a two-pronged attack. On one prong, you and your scientific friends con-

---

[17]A blood culture is a simple procedure wherein a small amount of blood from the patient is added to a medium that will promote the growth of any bacteria that may be living in the bloodstream. The bacteria then may be identified and the appropriate antibiotic chosen for treatment.

tinue to do your best to discover whatever regularities there appear to be in nature, and let my friends, the psychiatrists and other clinicians, decide if attention to these regularities offers any hope of improved treatment effectiveness. On the other prong, what I suggest for them is a treatment-based approach that goes something like this. Given that I have treatments A, B, C, D, E, and F in my arsenal, what I want to know about my patients is the benefit and the risk of applying each treatment. Any facts that I find to be useful in these considerations are welcome; my concern being to improve my batting average.[18]

In fact, I believe that the process of (1) finding a promising treatment (usually a logical process based on laboratory, non-human research), (2) refining the criteria for selecting candidates for the treatment through serial clinical trials, and (3) refining the treatment based on observations made during these trials is a scientific approach that has little to do with reliability of diagnosis. At the risk of pedantry, let me again say that any set of categories, for that matter any "language," is only as good as it is useful; that is, as it serves human ends. Why don't you talk with an academic clinician about this?

Inquirer: I certainly will.

---

[18]We will hope he and his colleagues keep track of this batting average. There exists a widespread human tendency to remember one's successes and forget one's failures. Recall the historical example of the practice of bloodletting in medicine discussed in Dialogue I, "The Young Psychiatrist."

Dialogue III

THE ACADEMIC CLINICIAN

T HE Academic Clinician runs a ward in a teaching psychiatric hospital. His job is to diagnose and treat patients in a manner that serves as a model example to professionals in training. He engages in little research or investigative activities. He does not appear burned out.

Academic Clinician:	Say there. I'd like a few words with you.
Inquirer:	Most certainly.
Academic Clinician:	I've just come from an interesting session with one of my psychiatric colleagues who seems upset by something you said about diagnosis in psychiatry.
Inquirer:	I know whom you mean. All I said in short was that while there may well be clusters of qualities that characterize people who seek psychiatric help, psychiatrists have as yet failed to develop a procedure whereby an individual's membership in one cluster as opposed to another can be reliably decided.
Academic Clinician:	In other words, diagnosis in psychiatry is unreliable, has limited validity, and in general leads to little new understanding.
Inquirer:	Fairly right.
Academic Clinician:	You know, running a psychiatric ward and supervising trainees in psychiatry is hard enough without all you Ibsenian prophets pestering my residents with your claims of the ideal. In clincial practice, Brand notwithstanding, the devil is *not* compromise; the devil is indecision. Physicians need to act, and for action, conviction rather than certainty is enough. At

Inquirer:

some point, the philosophical issues have been debated long enough and it's time to do something. But surely the problem of diagnosis does arise. How do you respond to sincere inquiry by confused trainees?

Academic Clinician:

I tell my house staff that diagnosis in psychiatry serves two purposes. First, third-party payers need some assurance that "unnecessary services" aren't being provided. Look at DSM-III, the official organ of the psychiatric party. Under the "atypical" subcategory of most of the major diagnoses, you could place any person with any complaint that happens to contain emotional terms. In this sense, diagnosis is a silly game that all doctors, not just psychiatrists, play with insurance companies.

Inquirer:

Don't you feel at all dishonest doing that?

Academic Clinician:

Hell no! Our patients are sick, and what we do for them helps a lot. In fact, it probably saves the insurance companies ten dollars for every one they lay out. I'd love to have a good diagnostic scheme as long as it allowed room for everyone who genuinely needs help. But, until it arrives, I'm not going to deny help to sick persons, or drive them into fiscal despair, because of our inadequacies.

Inquirer:

I see. The moral principle here is something like "the intent of the insurance company is to provide coverage for its clients when they genuinely need it, and technicalities should not be allowed to impede this coverage."

Academic Clinician:

Something like that. Anyway, we pick the best diagnostic category assignment we can. What else can be asked of us?

Inquirer:

And purpose number two?

Academic Clinician:

Observation. In psychiatry, there are no laboratory tests yet that can be substituted for clinical awareness and understanding. We can't perform a perfunctory physical exam and then send the patient through an enormous battery of laboratory tests that make the diagnosis for us. Useful biochemical and physiological measures are being developed, to be sure, but no matter how many we get we will, *in principle*, still need to know our patients well. In the beginning, at least, trainees are motivated to develop this level of understanding of their patients partly by a need to "make a diagnosis."

Inquirer: What do you mean "in principle"? How do you know that some laboratory measure won't be developed that will make the entire business as precise as cardiology or endocrinology?[1]

Academic
Clinician: Laboratory measures may be helpful, but in the final analysis will never have the significance to the psychiatrist that they have to all other medical specialists. Before I get into this point in detail, I would like to touch on a few points about a more general topic, that is, the overall relationship between the practice of psychiatry and the practice of science. I think that this relationship limits the relevance of developments in taxonomy, or any other basic science, to clinical practice.

Inquirer: You are going to talk about the "art of medicine," aren't you, and about personal values?

Academic
Clinician: Oh, please, give me a bit more credit. Those pieties have been tramped through long enough. What I mean to communicate begins with an illustration. Assume I'm a physician engaged in pulmonary medicine; you're a patient complaining of difficulty

---

[1]Precision in most fields of medicine is often attributed in direct proportion to the reliance of the specialist on instrument diagnosis, the electrocardiograph being a classic example. However, consider this from Henry Marriott, an international expert in electrocardiographic diagnosis: "Too many people are limping their way through life maimed by the unkind cuts of electrocardiographic interpretation. . . . Remember these facts: the range of normal is wide and its limits cannot be satisfactorily defined. . . ." Sound familiar? See Marriott, Henry J. L.: *Practical Electrocardiography* (Baltimore, Williams & Wilkins Co., 1972).

breathing, and I've just completed a thorough workup of your complaints.

Inquirer: Okay.

Academic
Clinician: Now, what I have in my hand is a sheet of numbers that represent parameters of respiratory function. I have a measure of how much and how fast air moves out of your lungs, how much oxygen is in your blood, how many red cells there are, etc. To determine my intervention, I merely check all these numbers against the "range of normal." If they're abnormal, I treat and I modify my treatment until all or most of the numbers are in the range of normal. Notice that the term *normal* in this context refers to a numerical range that is determined empirically, that is, by measuring each parameter in large numbers of persons who are apparently free of disease with respect to this parameter. "This is an abnormal reading" is intended to be a statement of fact arrived at through accepted processes of observation and measurement by men whose motives are pure and whose methods are sound.[2]

Inquirer: So far so good. But what if, after treatment, all the numbers are back to "normal," but I still complain of difficulty breathing?

Academic
Clinician: Aha! You're anticipating me, but well and good. Of course, in that case, after appropriate rechecking, when I'm convinced there is no "organic basis" for your complaint, I refer you to a psychiatrist. Interestingly, the judgment that it is not normal to complain of difficulty in breathing when one's physiology is intact contains an equivocation on the term normal that often escapes notice. Normal in this context threatens to slip out of the realm of empirical fact and into the realm of social behavior. I'm really saying, "You shouldn't do that," rather than "To complain

---

[2]Our Academic Clinician is very academic. He is lucky in that medical research has already given him these normal ranges. He seems to be ignoring what was discussed in Dialogue II about observer variation, even in medicine.

when things appear all right is a statistically deviant behavior." In order to carry any empirical meaning, the latter statement would have to be based upon research generated data that are not presently available and will probably never be available.

The question we would need the answer to is, How many people who feel that they are in circumstances like those you feel you are in continue to complain? The answer may well be "all of them," in which case your behavior *is* normal. But, to close the circle, only intimate, personal knowledge of someone allows an observer to appreciate what a person feels his circumstances to be, and then make factually normative statements about that person's behavior.[3]

Inquirer: So psychiatrists must make normative judgments as if they had the results of such faultless research?

Academic
Clinician: Correct! Psychiatrists must have a notion of what thoughts, feelings, impulses, perceptions, and behaviors are normal and must be able to recognize deviations from these norms. These recognitions may be expressed as "value judgments," but they're not arbitrary value judgments, and they are certainly not based on arbitrary norms.

Inquirer: Then what norms are used?

Academic
Clinician: Those generated by the process of therapy itself! Habermas has made a valuable contribution in this area, especially with his theory of communicative competence.[4] I will try to summarize the main ideas. The goal of the process of therapy is the creation of an "ideal speech situation." In such a situation, therapist and patient may arrive, by a process of discourse, at mutually recognized norms whose claim to validity

---

[3]He adds a view of normality to those considered in Dialogue II. The problem will reappear in Dialogue VIII, "The Psychiatric Scientist."

[4]See Habermas, J.: What is universal pragmatics? *Communication and the Evolution of Society* (Boston, Beacon Press, 1979). Habermas is a contemporary German philosopher in the hermeneutic tradition. See also Gadamer, H.G.: *Truth and Method* (New York, Seabury Press, 1975.). There will be more on hermeneutics — the interpretation of signs — in Dialogue VI, "The Mind Scientist."

rests upon the therapist and patient's mutual awareness of the rationality of the process that generated them. So I don't "help you become normal," rather I conduct myself in a way that allows you, if you will, to recognize, criticize, reject, and correct your own thoughts, beliefs, predispositions, expectations, and actions in the context of a normative structure that you and I create. To do otherwise is not to conduct therapy, but to coerce.[5]

Inquirer: Yes, but norms could arise in a situation like that which are totally out of step with the norms of the "outside world" — the patient would be worse off than if he tried to conform to "popular" conventional norms.

Academic
Clinician: Agreed. Part of the job of the therapist is to represent those norms as he understands them, along with his assessment of the consequences of behaving according to different norms. That is part of his contribution to the discourse.

Inquirer: You are making sense, but you're referring now mainly to the "talking" aspect of therapy, aren't you?

Academic
Clinician: Correct. I am referring to the exchange of meanings via linguistic symbols. Of course, there is a lot more to psychiatry these days. You may be wondering about the other aspects of psychiatric treatment and how their deployment is determined by the diagnostic scheme.

Inquirer: I am indeed. So far we've established that the background of your interventions, that is, your "biological" interventions if I may borrow a popular term, is an ongoing symbolically mediated social interaction wherein the thoughts, feelings, and conduct of the patient are systematically studied with

---

[5]The Academic Clinician is diverging into the area of therapy, which is not our main concern here. Because he does develop a communicating relationship with his patients involving an exchange of signs, the Inquirer is willing to allow the intermezzo and join the digression for awhile. As promised, signs and their interpretation will become a major topic of discussion later.

reference to norms that begin as "popular" norms but become unique creations of the therapeutic relationship.

Academic
Clinician: Right. Now, you say, what about medications, electroconvulsive treatment, sleep deprivation, biofeedback, and the like?

Inquirer: Yes, the so-called *somatic therapies*. After reading a recent textbook of psychopharmacology, I am wondering if disordered brain physiology underlies all psychiatric illness. It sure seems like we're on the edge of having useful laboratory tests based on disordered physiology![6]

Academic
Clinician: Beyond the edge! Today we can look at several dozen chemical values in blood, urine, saliva, and cerebrospinal fluid, reflecting endocrine function, neurotransmitter function and mineral regulation; we can measure brain waves asleep and awake with highly sophisticated computer programs that read data in ways totally unanticipated by the old clinicians. We can measure intellectual function, social behavior, reflexes, psychomotor performance, and a host of other physiological and behavioral parameters with undreamed of precision, accuracy, and reproducibility. Moreover, we can provoke all of these chemical and

---

[6]See Maas, J. W.: Clinical implications of pharmacological differences among antidepressants. In Lipton, M. A., DiMascio, A., and Killam, K. F. (Eds.): *Psychopharmacology: A Generation of Progress* (New York, Raven Press, 1978, p. 955) for discussion of how challenges with pharmacologic agents can be used to classify psychiatric patients. Electrical events in the brain are also useful (see Goodin, D. S., Squires, K. C., and Starr, A.: Long latency event-related components of the auditory evoked potential in dementia (*Brain 101*:635, 1978), and Coble, P., Foster, F. G., and Kupfer, D. J.: Electroencephalographic sleep diagnosis of primary depression (*Archives of General Psychiatry, 33*:1124, 1976), as are urinary and blood chemistries (see Fawcett, J., Maas, J., and DeKirmenjian, H.: Depression and MHPG excretion (*Archives of General Psychiatry, 26*:246, 1972). Patterns of labeled glucose-analog uptake in whole, living brain, which can now be visualized by emission-computed tomography, are also being used to identify psychiatric illness. See Buchsbaum, M.S., Ingvar, D.H., Kessier, R., et al: Cerebral glucography with positron tomography: use in normal subjects and in patients with schizophrenia (*Archives of General Psychiatry, 251*:9, 1982).

behavioral systems with various stimuli and appreciate response characteristics that would be missed without provocation.

Using combinations of these measures we can distinguish categories and subcategories of psychiatric syndromes from each other and from normals. The beauty of this type of classification is that the critical features are "objective" (i.e they are based on direct observation of pointer readings and therefore lead to high diagnostic reliability).

Inquirer: But are we sure that we know what categories based on these characteristics mean?

Academic
Clinician: There's the rub! In some cases they mean that the clinician can expect differences in prognosis and treatment response. In some cases they predict and retrodict family history. In other cases we don't yet know what they mean.

Inquirer: So, psychiatrists may yet be able to abandon clinical signs and symptoms altogether and diagnose patients in the laboratory.

Academic
Clinician: No. Practically, it is because all of these laboratory tests are significantly less than 100 percent sensitive and specific. As far as these test results go, some patients look like normals and some look like patients. Besides, we can't test everybody for everything, so we are required to use signs and symptoms in order to identify who to test and how to interpret the test results. For example, it is now well established that about 50 percent of individuals suffering from major depressive illness have an abnormal endocrine response to a test dose of dexamethasone, a powerful steroid hormone. Because only 4 percent of normals have this abnormal response, the observation of this response in a depressed patient should be evidence that depressive illness is the correct

diagnosis.[7] But clinical signs and symptoms are still needed to determine whom to test! What would an abnormal test mean in a well individual?

Laboratory tests are also of limited value in psychiatry *in principle*. Consider the following scenario: It is 1988 and we have determined that all persons who complain of suicidal depression have an elevated serum uranium, and no person who does not feel suicidally depressed has an elevated uranium. We have the perfect lab test: 100 percent specificity and sensitivity. Now imagine that someone comes to see a psychiatrist and says he feels suicidally depressed but his serum uranium is normal. What does the psychiatrist do then? Refuse to help the individual? Perhaps the neurosurgeon can say to the patient, "You may be ill but I find no neurosurgical condition and therefore cannot treat you," but the psychiatrist cannot. The psychiatrist is precisely that physician who is responsible for the "residual" patient, the one who fits no category. The psychiatrist can say, "I find no evidence of disease X in you," but he cannot say, "Your suffering does not deserve treatment." Lab tests may determine the *type* of treatment but will never be adequate to classify all of the patients that psychiatrists properly treat.

Inquirer: The best that could be expected appears to be that some percentage of patients could be precisely classified, with treatment based upon their diagnostic category; the unclassifiable ones will require treatment determined in another way, possibly by differential weighing of signs and symptoms versus personality traits versus circumstances, or some similar process.

Academic
Clinician: Correct. And this is why psychiatry will always be

[7]Carroll, B. J., Feinberg, M., Greden, J. F., Tarika, J., Albala, A. A., Haskett, R. F., James, N. M., Kronfol, Z., Lohr, N., Steiner, M., de Vigne, J. P., and Young, E.: A special laboratory test for the diagnosis of melancholia. (*Archives of General Psychiatry 38*:15, 1981). Also see Spar, J. and Larue, A.: Major depression in the elderly: DSM-II criteria and the dexamethasone suppression test as predictors of treatment response (*American Journal of Psychiatry*, 1983 in press).

more than whatever the scientists think it is, will always entail some judgments that cannot be intersubjectively validated, and will probably always be tentative, inefficient, and costly. We deal with lives and histories which have trajectories through a life space. Ortega said, "Man has no nature, only a history." He was incorrect; we have both. Psychiatrists, in addition to being psychobiological engineers, must be "historians of the individual," revisionist historians at that. Diagnosis, then, can only be a relevant aspect of psychobiological engineering, and this can only "improve" psychiatric practice to a limited degree.[8]

Inquirer: In a way, you suggest the relationship of psychiatry to medicine is like that of philosophy to science. That is, as soon as a problem in philosophy is seen to be solvable, usually as a result of some technological advance, it ceases to be part of the province of philosophy and becomes part of science. Space used to be a problem for philosophy: now it is a problem for physics. So with psychiatry, or so it seems. Helping people by talking to them may work, but it is a personal, subjective, inefficient process. To the extent that the same symptoms become accessible to non-symbolic intervention, for example, a drug, they potentially become a part of medicine and lost to psychiatry.

Academic
Clinician: Perhaps. The examples of general paresis, myxedema madness, and normal pressure hydrocephalus are outstanding. But I will always maintain that *psychoactive* drug treatment should be conducted by psychiatrists who talk with and know their patients. Psychiatric illness is a realm of human misery that finds its expression in language and has, therefore, an *interpersonal* forum. Accordingly, the risks of abuse are partially contained. Lionel Trilling once said, "We must be aware

---

[8]Practitioners as craftsmen tend to be dogmatic about what "always" will be and what "cannot" and what "must be" done. This stance probably arises from their daily task of making important life and death decisions about peoples' lives. Since these decisions are seldom challenged, practitioners seem more assured than the rest of us.

of the dangers which lie in our most generous wishes. Some paradox of our nature leads us, when once we have made our fellow men the objects of our enlightened interest, to go on to make them the objects of our pity, then our wisdom, ultimately of our coercion."[9]

Inquirer: In fact, with the psychiatrist's privileged access to scientific knowledge of human behavior, he is already in a position to be fairly coercive. After all, patients don't know enough to evaluate the treatment they receive. In that sense, they are victims and may be "linguistically free" in the therapeutic hour, but biochemically strait-jacketed. I appreciate that the relationship between human freedom and the facticity of the organism is a complex one, but surely manipulation of the organism can at least limit the freedom of the individual. How do you avoid this?

Academic
Clinician: By insisting that the patient take part in each decision. Nowhere does informed consent play a bigger role than it does here. The psychiatrist must educate the patient about the state of the art of whatever treatment approach will be used. This includes estimates of expected benefits as well as expected costs. Then the patient chooses.

Inquirer: Sounds good, but in practice I can't believe that you could ever know those facts with adequate reliability, let alone communicate them to a patient.

Academic
Clinician: To that all I can say is we do the best we can and acknowledge that our discussion ends on an appropriate note, once again underscoring the fiduciary nature of the relationship between not only patient and doctor, but clinician and scientist. I must trust the reliability of the work of basic and clinical scientists, and the patient must trust the reliability of my judgment. There is no escaping personal responsibility for any of these

---

[9]Cited in Didion, J: *Slouching Towards Bethlehem* (New York, Dell Publishing Co., 1968, pp. 161-162).

decisions; the scientists must decide which data to publish, I must decide which data to believe, the patient must decide which doctor to patronize.

Polanyi said it well: "Science can never be more than an affirmation of certain things we believe in. These beliefs must be adopted responsibly, with due consideration of the evidence and with a view to universal validity. But eventually they are ultimate commitments, issued under the seal of our personal judgment. At some point we shall find ourselves with no other answer to queries than to say, "Because I believe so." That is what no set of rules, or any model of science based on a system of rules, can do; it cannot say, "Because I believe so." Only a person can believe something, and only I myself can hold my own beliefs. For the holding of these I must bear the ultimate responsibility; it is futile, and I think also ignoble, to hunt for systems and machines which will take that burden from me. . . ."[10] I have quoted a number of philosophers here, especially in areas of value and views of the world. Why don't you talk to a philosopher who knows something about world views and metaphysics?

Inquirer: I shall.

---

[10]See Polanyi, M.: *Psychological Issues*, Vol. 6, No. 4 (New York, International Universities Press, 1974).

THE METAPHYSICIAN

T HE Metaphysician is not a physician, nor is he meta to physicians. He is a well-rounded philosopher who specializes in metaphysics. He is a professorial-looking fellow with long wispy hair, thick glasses and a faraway gleam in his eye.

Metaphysician: Why come to me? I don't know anything about psychiatry and its problems.

Inquirer: The Academic Clinician suggested that metaphysics is ultimately involved in our domain of psychiatry. Metaphysics is concerned with world views. The world views of psychiatry may relate to its fundamental problem of classifying its subject matter. I gather that classification is a matter of dividing up, or arranging, or clustering into kinds the objects of inquiry in a field. How it is done may depend to some extent on how people define the objects and choose to view the world made up of them.

Metaphysician: Agreed. But watch out when you start talking about "THE WORLD." Before we get to that, what does psychiatry take as its objects or kinds of objects of inquiry?

Inquirer: Without defining what an object is, I would say that psychiatry's objects are people with complaints of certain kinds of troubles who show signs and symptoms of what we call mental disorders. This answer may not be too helpful to you because we have lots of our own troubles in defining mental disorders, let alone grouping them into reliable categories.

Metaphysician: Before we get to your *Menschanschauung*, let us consider your *Weltanschauung*. There are many ways to view, describe, picture or represent

41

"THE WORLD." It sounds like psychiatrists entertain some version of realism in which it is assumed there exists a real world out there consisting of objects independent of ourselves as observers, but not necessarily independent of *any* observer. A psychiatrist's task is to understand certain undesirable aspects of this world, such as mental disorders, in order to reduce or prevent or eliminate them through active interventions. You are involved in not just viewing a world, but the view becomes a determinant of how you will *act* in that world as professional experts.[1]

Inquirer: I think most psychiatrists would endorse that view even though they may have never asked themselves about it in the ennobled terms of "metaphysics."

Metaphysician: Let me start with a few elementary points. First, consider your own personal everyday experience, the realm of pure sensation. You see two-dimensional patches of color and hear sounds from various directions, that is, you receive signs. This experience of receiving signs becomes described fact when we use words to communicate it. Described fact, because it involves words, is brought under terms designating con-

---

[1]There are various kinds of metaphysical beliefs in realism ranging from naive realism (a belief that we directly observe the world) to transcendental realism (belief in a transobservational real). They share the view that there is "something that is out there" independent of ourselves although known only through ourselves. That is, there exists no "absolute" reality. What we call "reality" is a metaphysical assignment relativized to our values as humans. Peirce believed we know the "not us out there" through signs of which we are their interpreters (cf. Dialogue I, note 19). For a treatment of modern transcendental realism, see Bhaskar, R.: *A Realist Theory of Science*, (Leeds, Leeds Books, 1975). This version of realism involves the construction and testing of models of the transobservational real, a topic which will be of concern in Dialogue VI, "The Mind Scientist." For an extensive defense of the realist position, see Boyd, R.: Scientific realism and naturalistic epistemology. In Asquith, P. D., and Giere, R. (Eds.): *Proceedings of the 1980 Biennial Meeting of the Philosophy of Science Associations* (East Lansing, Philosophy of Science Association, 1981, vol. II, p. 613). For the empiricist counter, see Van Frassen, B. C.: Theory construction and experiment: an empiricist view (p. 663 in the same volume, 1981) as well as his *The Scientific Image* (Oxford, Clarendon, 1980).

cepts and, eventually, theories.[2] Described fact involves external objects which realists take to be independent of them. If you are a realist, you believe our real "world" consists of differentiated individual objects (i.e. entities, items, things or processes) with properties that change over time. Objects can be factual or conceptual, and a concept can be about another concept. Our conceptual objects are human constructs, which serve human purposes in our interactions with this real world, including other humans and their concepts.

There are three further points to keep in mind. First, the individual factual objects of our world are indefinite. For example, is a man with one leg still a man? How many parts can you subtract and still call a man a "man"? Second, conceptual classes of empirically observable objects are inexact, having hazy boundaries. Since the properties defining the class may have quantitative variations, it may be difficult to decide whether an individual belongs to a class or not. We decide on boundaries and pretend more or less exact classes for our own purposes when we construct theories, laws, and general principles. Third, the perceptible world consists of continua which we relentlessly render up to suit ourselves. When does a day begin? We are line-drawers. Where do we draw the line between California and Nevada? Between the hand and

---

[2]See Russell, B.: *Our Knowledge of the External World* (London, Allen and Unwin, 1952). It was Russell who also noted that no philosopher doubts the existence of an objective reality while holding a crying baby in his arms in the middle of the night. See also Professor W. Allen's essay "My Philosophy" in *Getting Even* (New York, Random House, 1966). "Is there anything out there? And why? And must they be so noisy? Finally, there can be no doubt that one characteristic of 'reality' is that it lacks essence. That is not to say it has no essence, but merely lacks it. (The reality I speak of here is the same one Hobbes described, but a little smaller)."

the wrist?[3] Thus, what is called the "real world" consists *in part* of our makings as well as our takings. The term *fact* comes from the Latin "facere," which means "to make." William James had a neat way of putting it: "The *that* of a thing is its own, but the *what* depends on the *which* and the *which* depends on *us*."

Inquirer:

Is it that "us" you were alluding to when earlier you warned me about talk of "THE WORLD"?

Metaphysician:

Yes, indeed. The realist talks about "THE WORLD" as if there were one system out there which is the same for all observers. But his observer is human and his reference frame is human-centered. One could imagine different sorts of observers such as organisms that have only "feelers" as sensing organs, or organisms that can respond to sound waves far beyond our range of perception, or organisms like some insects which can see by infrared light to which we are oblivious. To these observers, "THE" world is very different from ours since they are receiving different signs. So when we say the world, we must be clear about *whose* world; what world ver-

---

[3]See Körner, S.: *Experience and Theory* (New York, Humanities Press, 1966). Our world of immediate experience is churning, blurry, and run-together. When we describe classes of individuals who resemble one another according to shared properties, the resemblance class is inexact because we cannot always decide whether an individual belongs in, on the edge of, or outside the class. But when we create theories about these classes, we replace inexact empirical classes with the idealization of exact theoretical classes so that inferences rules can be applied. Körner makes clear that these inference rules in science are not strictly deductive. They do not necessarily involve the refinements of deductive calculi or even a two-valued logic. They may be partly deductive but they often utilize the ordinary verbal arguments with semantic and pragmatic entailments of material implication. The inference rules of material implication allow the p and q of p → q to be any propositions and the arrowed connection to be any relation as long as ¬ (p and ¬ q).

The working scientist knows all the time that he is using approximation procedures in making rough inductive inferences about inexact classes. His "logic" involves approximations as much as do his "measurements." Hence, the inferences of science take the form "if my hypothesis holds, then the empirical observations will probably, or will likely, or will tend to be such and such to some order of approximation." The replacement of a description of experience by an idealization of it is the price we pay for the power, the economy, and efficiency of simplifying inferences. In addition to the problem of inexact empirical classes, psychiatry must deal with the problem of polythetic classes as "The Biological Scientist" will explain in Dialogue V.

	sion for what set of equivalent observers.
Inquirer:	Don't we really perceive the world?
Metaphysician:	Once in Industan, according to a famous poem by John C. Saxe, based on a Jainist story, there were six wise, but blind, men who investigated an elephant. One stumbled into its side and said the elephant was very like a wall. Another, feeling the tusk, said it was rather like a spear. The third, holding the elephant's trunk, compared it to a snake, while the fourth, with his arms around the animal's foreleg, said it resembled a tree. The fifth heard sounds and felt the wind of a flapping ear so he declared the elephant to be a fan. The last wise man said the beast had the form of a rope since he took hold of its tail.

The moral for us is supposed to be that each was partially right and all were in the wrong. But were they? Those who think they see a whole elephant arrogantly declare them wrong. But is vision to be the final authority? If you think so, you should see a stage magician at least once a year. Our world is full of optical illusions (See Fig. 1). What we see is just as partial, incomplete, and biased as what the blind men felt and heard. Signs are always incomplete. We do not see an elephant; we get only a view of an elephant. It is simply a shorthand of language to say that we see an elephant, or hear one, or feel one, or smell one.[4] These abbreviations stand for perceptual judgments in which we get a view *of*, a sound *of*, a feel *of*, a smell *of*. Our perceptions

---

[4]For an early articulation of this perspective realism, see Ortega y Gasset: *The Origin of Philosophy* (New York, W. W. Norton, 1967). In 1943 Ortega wrote, "According to a popular expression, we would say that the 'aspect' is the 'face shown' by reality. Reality puts it on us.[6] (Ortega's reference 6: "And, in fact, in lieu of 'aspect,' one could justifiably endow the word *face* with terminological value in ontology.") If it were possible to integrate the countless 'aspects' of a thing, we would be able to fathom the thing itself, for the thing is the 'entirety.' Since this is impossible, we must be content with possessing merely 'aspects' of the thing and not the thing itself — as Aristotle and Saint Thomas believed."

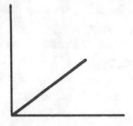

Figure 1. When you look at this two-dimensional drawing of three simple lines, do you see (a) an intersected right angle; (b) a cube from above with its corner pointing towards you; (c) a cube from below with its corner pointing away; or (d) something else?

represent the domain of OF.[5]

We communicate with one another and ourselves about objects only under particular descriptions. Peirce maintained a man's essential life was made up of his communings both with others and himself. We commune with signs. The signs we receive are information structures carrying many pieces of information. We, as interpreters of the signs, assign meaning to aspects of the signs by categorizing them into multiple classes and converting them into beliefs. The output descriptions used in communings express the construals of a category framework. The converse domain of OF, the "real" items, have an ontological status independent of our knowledge of them.

Our knowledge of objects is always partial, patchy, provisional, and defeasible. As Peirce said, signs stand for something, to someone, *only in some respect*. When we say our knowledges are "true," we mean they are adequate/inadequate, reliable/unreliable, useful/nonuseful, correct/ incorrect, informative or simply valuable commodities for human purposes. They help us enlarge and correlate the deliverances of an expanding human experience. Aristole remarked we move

[5]See Woodger, J. H.: *Biology and Language* (Cambridge, Cambridge University Press, 1950). Woodger was a biologist, logician, and thinker of commanding gifts. He also wrote the best monograph on medical psychology, entitled *Physics, Psychology and Medicine* (Cambridge, Cambridge University Press, 1956).

Inquirer:

Metaphysician:

from what is basic in us to what is basic in reality. But isn't there just one world looked at from different perspectives?

The difference may make a big difference in what is to be called "reality" and how one is to act in it. Let's assume events represent the changes of objects in some four-dimensional space-time manifold we call a world. A system capable of being activated by certain event patterns will resonate to these event patterns. The resonance Peirce termed the "interpretant" is determined by the signs received by an interpreter. The receiving system will prefer and derive "satisfaction" from certain patterns of informational event arrangements and not others. A system with different resonance capacities would read a different message from the events, or select a different set of events to read, because it uses a different code.[6]

A code is a set of rules whereby messages are converted from one representation to another. A code selects some events as signs and ignores others.[7] What is a signal or sign to us as human

---

[6]See Jauch, J. M.: *Are Quanta Real?* (Bloomington, Indiana University Press, 1973). It is noteworthy that this delightful book on quantum theory is in dialogue format. Notice the Metaphysician's introduction of the affective term *satisfaction*. Affective factors, such as cognitive and pragmatic satisfactions, are involved in scientific as well as philosophical inquiry, as will crop up repeatedly in dialogues to come.

[7]Some terminological clarification may be helpful here in following these information-theoretic concepts. A *signal* is the physical form of a sign carrying information. It can be light waves, sound waves, vibrations, etc. Information is neutral, having no meaning or significance by itself. Recall (Dialogue I note 19) that a sign has as a source an object that it represents, which is taken in some respect (its properties or ground), determining or creating an interpretant in an interpreter who receives the sign. The signal is a physical vehicle for a *message*, the information-content of the sign as determined by an orderly selection of signs. The message, physically embodied in the signal, acquires significance or meaning for a receiver when internal patterns of constructs, interpretants, that fit the orderly messages in the sign, activate, sustain or produce beliefs of unique semantic content. See Dretske, F. I.: *Knowledge and the Flow of Information* (Cambridge, MIT Press, 1981).

When an interpreter responds to a sign by producing a unique interpretant, this interpretant constitues a *new* type of sign having significance and stands in the same triadic relation of object-ground-interpretant to the same object as did the initial triggering sign. Thus, sign types become associated with a working system of other sign types that undergoes progressive development through a potentially endless series. (We did not call Peirce the Thinker's Thinker for nothing. For some peculiar nineteenth century reasons like getting a divorce from

→

may be noise to some other observer-actor and conversely. Codes are not absolute. There may be several messages read from the same patterns of information processes. Which one is "real," which one is "correct"? Maybe they all are correct in some sense since they are relative to, and parochial to, the interests of different observer-actors. This is what I think James meant: what we call "reality" is that which is real for us as human, as one of the kinds of observer-actor using a particular "natural" code which we assume derived from a biological evolutionary process operating over a long time. The workings of a world are read off this model. I hope this is not all getting too abstruse.

Inquirer: I think I follow you dimly. What you call a model is equivalent to a set of Peirce's interpretants, a system of representations with semantic content.

Metaphysician: Quite so. Let me draw you a simple diagram to visualize the points made thus far.[8] Suppose the object is an apple (See Fig. 2). Light waves reflected from the apple constitute sign events or signs. They are received by an interpreter in whom they activate an interpretant, a construal such that the object is identified as an apple. In

---

a woman with family connections to Harvard and marrying a *French* woman, Peirce was never able to obtain a tenured university position. He made a living by working for the U.S. Coastal and Geodetic Survey!) If the universe is made up of signs, as Peirce thought, then, in a current idiom, the basic "stuff" of the universe consists of virtual and actual information processes having degrees of activity. Information processes bunched into clumps and hardened into tradition, we call things or objects; information processes well-spread-out we call a field or space-time. It is certainly easier to understand how molecules could derive from active information processes than vice versa.

This view comes close to the epistemology of many contemporary quantum theorists such as David Bohm who differentiates between an implicate order of information and the explicate order of observable objects. See Bohm, D.: *Wholeness and the Implicate Order* (London, Routledge and Kegan Paul, 1980), and Davies, P.: *Other Worlds: A Portrait of Nature in Rebellion: Space, Superspace, and the Quantum Universe* (New York, Simon and Schuster, 1980). If you can tolerate the Zen that goes along for the ride, see Zukav, G.: *The Dancing Wu Li Masters: An Overview of the New Physics* (New York, Bantam, 1979). What all this has to do with modern psychiatry will be unfolded in future dialogues. A slight hint of relevance appears in the Metaphysician's final statement about skewed interpretants in this dialogue.

[8]He draws Figure 2 on the blackboard in the background.

modern terms, we say the external signs, through energy transduction, become mapped into, or encoded into, the relevant portions of a model.

What we call coded model representation is quite similar to Peirce's interpretants.

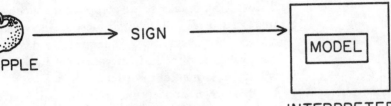

Figure 2. The internal model, carried by the interpreter, consists of a network of concepts, conceptual structures, and construals.

Inquirer: You said the apple was an object that somehow gave off sign events by reflecting light waves that we pick up. But what is the apple itself apart from its signs?

Metaphysician: Now you are becoming a real metaphysician. What are the ultimate stuffs or objects of the world that constitute both the us and the not-us? Our grasp or construal of an object we can call a conceptual object involving universals or properties, categories by which we individuate and characterize a factual object out there, a not-us. But what is the factual object "really" like? Perhaps it itself is just another sign event and the universe consists of an endless series of evolving sign events, one acting on the other. But this is getting too far away from your psychiatric problem, namely, people with construals or internal models that are in some way aberrant. Your factual objects are people with aberrant conceptual objects.

Inquirer: Right. A person who has a model of his experience is part of our factual problem world. In psychiatry, our objects of inquiry are ill people who carry certain representations or interpretants

	or construals that trouble them.
Metaphysician:	If you wish, you can speak of a physical state of physical systems and conceptual states of conceptual systems as long as you remember that conceptual structures in human heads are still properties or states of a particular physical individual. Since classes are components of conceptual structures, the main question is whether classes you construct are adequate to deal with the problems of a field, in your case individuals who possess mental disorders.
Inquirer:	In their own conceptual models, psychiatrists have some sort of construals of patients possessing aberrant concepts or beliefs and are convinced classes of such patients can be formed. How can we justify this conviction?
Metaphysician:	A few more terms may help to get us under way. The term *ontology* means the study of what actually exists in what, for convenience, let us henceforth call "the world." Epistemology signifies the study of our knowledge about the world. If you say there *are* classes of patients, you must be careful about the sense of the term *are*. Remember, we said classes are human constructs. People contain a representation or conceptual model of what is, to them, their real world. The problem is how adequately this model of this real world fits, meshes, or accommodates to that which is the case, the that-which-is, in that world.
Inquirer:	It sounds like you are talking about a concept of truth.
Metaphysician:	Truth is a vexed and tangled tale in my field. There are many kinds of truths — logical, mathematical, philosophical, factual. I would think psychiatrists, like scientists, are interested primarily in factual truth, in that which is the case, for which there is good evidence, in their particular domain. How do we know when one of our assertions about what is the case is true?

Let me continue my distinction between ontology and epistemology. Let truth$_1$ represent what is really true ontically and let truth$_2$ represent our knowledge of truth$_1$.

Inquirer: By "what is really true ontically," of course, you mean "what really is," period, don't you? Truth$_1$ must be just what is, prior to any reading or interpretation of it. Truth$_2$ then is about truth$_1$ and is itself in a different ontological category.

Metaphysician: Yes. Truth$_1$ is not to be construed as something categorically similar but not quite the same as truth$_2$. You are correct; truth$_2$ is about truth$_1$ but truth$_1$ is not about anything; it just is. Truth$_2$, conceptual structures in our model of the world, are revisable, corrigible and improvable. We correct and adjust them over time through a historical and evolutionary process of problem solving. Truth$_2$ at t_0 can become false later at t_1. Another truth$_2$ takes its place to eventually be replaced by still another truth$_2$. Our hero here, Peirce, called it *contrite fallibilism*.[9]

Inquirer: Does this mean that what we now have as truth$_2$ is more true, that is, closer to truth$_1$, than what we had previously as truth$_2$?

Metaphysician: Some think of scientific progress as gaining on truth$_1$, whereas others think we cannot be gaining on something when we don't know where that something is to begin with or even what space is involved. While realists agree there is something out there besides ourselves, some realists believe our knowledge successively approximates this

---

[9]Again, cf. Peirce, *Collected Papers, 1,* p. 10. We must trust our own minds, believing at the same time in fallibilism, that is, that recognition of error is always and everywhere possible. Peirce remarked, "Only once, as far as I remember, in all my lifetime have I experienced the pleasure of praise — not for what it might bring but in itself. That pleasure was beatific, and the praise that conferred it was meant for blame. It was that a critic said of me that I did not seem to be *absolutely sure of my own conclusions.*" Cf. Gallie, W. B.: *Peirce and Pragmatism* (Middlesex, Penguin, 1952, p. 56). For elaborations on the distinctions between the two truths, see Brown, M. H. I.: *Perception, Theory and Commitment* (Chicago, Precedent, 1977).

"real" truth, whereas others are willing to settle for a modest empirical adequacy in dealing with the real. Scientists use the term *true* in a way different from philosophers and logicians. Scientific "truths" are conclusions that involve approximation procedures that, in turn, involve evaluative decision procedures on the part of each scientist. Does a theoretical prediction approximate an empirical observation to some adequate or satisfactory degree? Who decides? According to what decision rule? Perhaps scientific progress simply means we advance in a cumulative sense from what we now know to what we wish to know. Or maybe we also become a little more certain or a little clearer about the little we do know.[10]

Truth$_2$ has demonstrable utility in organizing and making coherent our ever-enlargening experiences. It is true enough, often enough over a range of applications. Truth$_2$ can, like the integers, increase but not converge on a finite value.

I notice that, according to physicists, gravity is

---

[10]If we continue the analogy of decoding and recoding the messages of a world consisting basically of active information processes, a progression of truth$_2$ means we successfully move farther along more and more patterns of messages of interest to us. Periodic recurrences are recognized in the patterns and we then recode them into descriptions or regularities called general "laws." A message may have more than one decoding, but as a successful decoding gets farther and farther along the patterned sequences, the number of correct solutions becomes greatly reduced and we can foresee, by extrapolation, the rest of the patterns we are engaged in. A crossword puzzle with only two-dimensional patterns, left-to-right and top-to-bottom, can be hard enough. But imagine an uncountable number of patterned messages in an *n*-dimensional space and you will grasp how difficult it all is. Science is self-improving and self-extending. Scientific knowledge and techniques improve, but whether the accumulated knowledge is "truer," we cannot say. We may be gaining on truth$_1$ as we increase our samples of the world, but if truth$_1$ is a million miles away and you are gaining on it a few feet a century, it doesn't make much difference. Our current models of the world, truth$_2$, are always imperfect, incomplete, ill-fitting, and blurred, partial matches, containing anomalies which we ignore, hoping they will be resolved eventually. Our beliefs are hoped-for truths; our best guesses for the time being. Truth$_2$ might fit truth$_1$ exactly but, being the way we are, we can never be sure. And truth$_1$ can change over time because the world evolves and develops. Properties of an object that are at one time lawfully associated may dissociate and no longer go together, as for example in a new strain of mutant bacteria. As the world evolves, new regularities and laws may emerge that were not present previously.

weakening and Hubble's constant is no longer constant. There is even some current doubt as to whether the speed of light is constant. Mathematics has lost its certainty.[11] Also, notice our everyday external world becomes greatly transformed, expanded, and differentiated, by human action. The processes of our world develop, effloresce, exfoliate, ramify, and evolve. Our experiences continuously expand, fan out, enlarge, and become clearer, more distinct and more differentiated. Caesar did not live in our current world. He could not know that his sword conducted electricity; nor could he have the experience of watching himself on television.

Inquirer:

The realist appears to be a modern scientist.

Metaphysician:

Not entirely. Some scientists are instrumentalists. They view theories as calculating devices, instruments for summarizing or systematizing the observed facts. They take the objects involved to be "as-if" metaphors. Other scientists, as realists, view the objects as literally true. Then there are mixtures of realism and instrumentalism in which what works is believed to do so because it is, in part, real.[12] Scientists are

---

[11]In the nineteenth century, when it became clear that science could not provide truth with certainty, as originally hoped, there was still a bastion of certainty in mathematics. But mathematical truth has also withered. For example, the Loewenheim-Skolem theory (1920-1933) demonstrated that an axiom system, designed to characterize a unique set of mathematical objects, does not do so; it can be assigned many interpretations. In 1931, Goedel showed that no mathematical system strong enough to generate arithmetic could be shown within itself to be consistent and that such systems are inescapably incomplete. For a masterful and thoroughly readable account of all this, see Klein, M.: *Mathematics: The Loss of Certainty* (New York, Oxford University Press, 1980). Another comprehensive treatment can be found in Davis, P.J., and Hersh, R.: *The Mathematical Experience* (Boston, Birkhause, 1981). For some fun and games with Goedel's theorems, see Hofstader, D.: *Goedel, Escher, Bach: An Eternal Golden Braid.* (New York, Basic Books, 1979).

[12]Einstein noted the opportunistic nature of scientists in respect to epistemologists. "No sooner has the epistemologist, who is seeking a clear system, fought his way through to such a system, that he is inclined to interpret the thought content of science in the sense of his system and to reject whatever does not fit into his system. The scientist, however, cannot afford to carry his striving for epistemological systematic that far. He accepts gratefully the epistemological conceptual analysis; but the external conditions, which are set for him by the

→

a peculiar breed. They seem to like to deny diversity. They try to explain the *many* in terms of the *one* and to reduce *becoming* to *being*. They begin searching for similarities, then after awhile call them equivalences or invariants, and wind up viewing them as identities. They deny change and try to abolish time. Perhaps this is why atemporal mathematical descriptions are so appealing to them.[13]

Inquirer: This might not be characteristic just of scientists but of human minds in general. It could be an example of what you mentioned earlier. Systems have certain abstracting categorizing operations that they use to interpret the informational processes of their world. The human mind, with its particular code derived through evolution, has a tendency to fix on some patterns as salient and not on others. It turns sources of event patterns, incomplete signs, into inferred items (things or processes) whose total quality it assumes to be constant. This may seem a peculiar strategy to philosophers, but it seems to be quite effective in anticipating events before they occur so that we can prevent them, or control them, or prepare ourselves for them, or control ourselves undergoing them.

---

facts of experience, do not permit him to let himself be too much restricted in the construction of his conceptual world by the adherence to an epistemological system. He must therefore appear to the systematic epistemologist as a type of unscrupulous opportunist; he appears as *realist* insofar as he seeks to describe a world independent of the acts of perception; as *idealist* insofar as he looks upon the concepts and theories as the free inventions of the human spirit (not logically derivable from what is empirically given); as *positivist* insofar as he considers his concepts and theories judified *only* to the extent to which they furnish a logical representation of relations among sensory experiences. He may even appear as *Platonist* or *Pythagorean* insofar as he considers the viewpoint of logical simplicity as an indispensable and effective tool of his research." See Einstein, A.: Reply to criticisms. In Schilpp, P. A. (Ed.): *Albert Einstein: Philosopher Scientist* (New York, Tudor, 1951, p. 684).

[13]He is alluding to Meyerson's Principle, which attempts to account for science in terms of a single overarching principle. The principle is a self-referent example in that it itself denies the diversity of the sciences and reduces the *many* to the *one*. See Zahar, E.: Einstein, Meyerson and the role of mathematics in physical discovery (*British Journal For the Philosophy of Science*, *31*:1, 1980).

Metaphysician: Granted and well-taken as a pragmatist. The
                  scientific realist has further presuppositions. He
                  assumes there is an overall uniformity, order,
                  harmony, pattern or design to an independent
                  world. The world of manifest experience is full of
                  turbulence and tumult, but underneath there is
                  an order to it. It is further posited there are two
                  loci of this order, that outside ourselves and that
                  which is symbolically represented in human ner-
                  vous systems. The realist cannot accept that the
                  independent world is chaotic, and he believes the
                  human mind itself is an ordered part of an
                  ordered world. Human nature is part of the
                  natural order.

                  A realist holds that there exists some sort of fit
                  or consonance between these two orderings. The
                  mind's ordering contains a re-coded model or
                  secondary representation of the first order code
                  that, to various degrees, fits or coordinates with
                  the way things are outside the mind. As a per-
                  sonal aside, it has always seemed to me very
                  strange that what we call the world has evolved in
                  such a way that it has been able to sever itself into
                  observing and observed parts. The human mind
                  is a part of the world that can observe part of the
                  world, including parts of the mind. Whatever is
                  observed about the world is only partially itself
                  and hence it will always partially elude itself. [14]

Inquirer: Why should we believe the world accessible to us
                  is ordered the way we think it is? It might be part-
                  ly chaotic or random, or it might be ordered ac-
                  cording to principles we are currently using. [15]

---

[14]It implies that the world has evolved subsystems that produce representations of itself.
Why? A very deep idea.

[15]Randomness and chaos are separate concepts. Automobiles may arrive at busy intersections
and customers may arrive at a store counter at random times during the day. The probability
of an individual arrival within any given time interval is not affected by individual arrivals in
other intervals. The whole set of individual arrivals has a probabilistic structure in that there
is a definite probability, in terms of a relative frequency, for a single arrival to occur within
→

Metaphysician: Although the world may at first appear to us as scattered mosaics, realists believe this world cannot be *entirely* chaotic (i.e. lawless) because the mind and its code is a product of nature, and he knows the mind is not entirely chaotic, although some of its processes at times seem to be (e.g. certain dreams). Parts of the world that we are not concerned with, and even parts of the mind, could be idiosyncratic and not lawful.[16] The human mind could not be completely and unlawfully chaotic because it is systematically and repeatedly successful in aiding humans to get what they want.

We do not just receive and interpret information-carrying signs; we act back on the sources of the signs to suit ourselves. In my diagram of Figure 2, I left out the action response of the in-

some time interval, such that predictions can be made according to a stochastic law. This sort of law does not state *which* car or customer will arrive; it does not dictate that any particular arrival occur among a set of independent individual arrivals. In contrast, chaos is lawless; it has no trends or probability measure at all. The independent world may be to a large extent stochastic and random, but it is not thereby chaotic or haphazard. See Bunge, M.: *Treatise on Basic Philosophy, Vol. 3, Ontology, I, The Furniture of the World* (Boston, Reidel, D., 1977, p. 208). Like that of information, the concept of probability is difficult to define even though we use it. Von Neuman said, "One does not understand things in mathematics — we just get used to them." The concept of probability will be further elucidated in Dialogue VIII with "The Psychiatric Scientist."

[16]The terms *law* and *lawful* have arisen a few times without comment. In a preliminary way, it should be remarked that the current concept of a scientific law has been considerably liberalized in contrast to the universal laws set up in classical mechanics. Laws of nature are not iron-clad pronouncements of a hand. They have not been whip-handed down by the red king or a shrouded law-giver. They do not dictate what is to happen, nor do they ordain what is to happen without exception throughout the whole universe and for all eternity. There is really only one universal law and that is "all laws except this one have exceptions." In modern parlance, laws are more like rules or directions or principles or instructions for navigating around in the world with some assurance about expectable events.

Law-like statements are descriptions of regular patterns. They themselves are not isomorphic to the patterns, only their meanings correspond to the patterns. In the description, "the chair is to the right of the table," the term *chair* is to the left of the word *table*. But from semantic knowledge, you know where the chair is relative to the table. If you follow a law or rule as an injunction, your behavior will accommodate to, or dovetail with, or fit the world in a mutual adaptation. Rules leave room for play and exceptions, uncharacteristic of the strict laws of classical mechanics. Laws and rules are impatient generalizations subject to modification in the light of further experience. There will be more on laws and rules in the dialogue with "The Mind Scientist."

terpreter only to keep things simple for a while. We interact with the world to get what we want. We intervene to get rid of what we do not want. By its interpretations the mind could not impose a radically different order on the world and still survive very long. Our semantic recodings of the world's patterns as laws must have some degree of accurate fit. The accuracy is demonstrated by the fact that we successfully correlate more and more experiences, anticipate events by foreseeing more clearly the rest of the patterns, and get where we want to go not only more efficaciously than in the past but more efficiently and more flexibly. A complete misreading of the messages would be a disaster for any living organism and maybe that is how some species became extinct. How is our own empirical utilitarian success possible? If that aspect of the world we are interested in were chaotic, our back actions would not give us what we want, except by accident. If the world were completely disordered, we wouldn't even realize it. Disorder is relative to an order. Notice also we do not always get what we want and things happen to us we do not want. The independent world is both partner and opponent for us. We must be chastened by the knowledge that what we term *objects* are things that object; they constitute an oppositional non-self, they are obdurate and they are not fully predictable and defeasible. If the world were unlawful having no regularities, we as humans would not be here to talk about it. There would be no such thing as minds at all, much less the products of science and technology which thus far represent humans' most powerful ways of intervening with the world to change it.[17]

Inquirer: We started talking metaphysics and now we are into science. Didn't the philosopher Popper assert

---

[17]See Rescher, N.: *Methodological Pragmatism: A Systems-Theoretic Approach to the Theory of Knowledge* (New York, New York University Press, 1977). This work provides a clear contemporary discussion of the pragmatic vantage point, which did not begin with the Americans Peirce and James, as popularly believed, but goes back at least to the Greek Sophists and Skeptics of 400-300 B.C.

there is a clear demarcation between science and metaphysics?[18]

Metaphysician: He did, but he is misunderstood on this point. He wanted to exclude fields he didn't like, like Marxism and psychoanalysis, from the imprimatur of "science." Popper is not opposed to the use of metaphysics in science. He wants to distinguish assertions which can be falsified from those which cannot.[19] The more useful distinction lies between science and pseudoscience. You and your colleagues will have to decide what is scientific and what is pseudoscientific psychiatry. Science is inescapably riddled with metaphysics under the guise of presuppositions. Woodger said any scientist who thinks he is above metaphysics is up to his neck in it. Presuppositions and world views are extremely important in steering scientific work. They may go unacknowledged, and they can unwittingly form the basis of many virulent scientific disputes. Russell concretely summarized one of the great arguments in physics: "Do you view the world as consisting of a bucket of molasses or as a pail of sand?" In one case a physicist will geometrize, in the others he will count. Neither yields a completely

---

[18]See Popper, K. R.: The demarcation between science and metaphysics. In Schilpp, P. A. (Ed.): *Philosophy of Rudolf Carnap* (Cambridge, Cambridge University Press, 1963). Also, cf. Popper, K. R.: *The Logic of Scientific Discovery* (New York, Basic Books, 1959).

[19]One cannot verify a universal statement of "all" (past, present and future) and one cannot falsify a singular statement because of the insufficiencies of observation. If you say, "there are no fish in this pond based on my fishing experience," it may be that you are a poor fisherman. Popper's view of science as running on falsification is too one-dimensional a view of scientific activity. Popperians would think baseball consists of striking out batters. See Weimer, W. B.: *Notes on the Methodology of Scientific Research* (Hillsdale, Erlbaum Associates, 1979).

Scientists do not intentionally labor to construct hypotheses for them to be destroyed by falsifications. Good hypotheses are cherished like children. Who wants one's children destroyed? When confronted by disconfirmatory evidence, hypotheses are modified, repaired and clung to for a long time before they are reluctantly let go. Because of errors of formulation, measurement errors, logical errors, small calculational errors accumulating at each step, and evaluative decisions about the acceptable degree of approximation in empirical observations, it may be just as difficult to refute a hypothesis as to confirm it. How does one establish that the refuting evidence is true if one can only falsify? For a lively discussion of the contrast between the way philosophers *view* science and the way scientists *do* science, see Wasserman, G. D.: *Brains and Reasoning: Brain Science As A Basis of Applied and Pure Philosophy* (London, Macmillan, 1974).

	satisfactory description.
Inquirer:	If people, members of our own human group, interpret or model the world in quite different ways, how do we know which is the correct model?
Metaphysician:	Recall that we do not perceive the items of our world at all in a direct way but only certain of their aspects through informational signs to which we assign a significance. Remember the six blind men and the elephant? Consider visual perception. As humans, we are capable of receiving only a very small band of wave forms within a broad electromagnetic spectrum. When the "raw" light waves to which humans are sensitive are reflected from an object and impinge on your retina, they initiate a progressive process of abstraction all along the way from retina to brain. The abstraction operations result in a loss of information from the input signs which are richer than the final product. A succession of multiple classifications is superimposed on the input waveforms, transduced from light waves to neural, electrochemical impulses. The final inter-pretation of the input you may label, for example, "sun," but the light waves you received left the sun eight minutes ago. For all you know, the sun may not even be there at this moment. What we "see" are final "readings," interpretations, construals or beliefs of unique semantic content that represent knowledge-acquisition achievements on our part.[20]

I will belabor the point. We do not just see, we see that an X is an object of a certain kind. When we say we perceive signs of spring, our saying is a shorthand way of saying we perceive signs *that* it is spring. Our internal representations are categorized and related to one another in the con-

---

[20]If one did not have an internal class for a visual sign, one would not "see" it at all. Cf. Hayek, F.A.: The primacy of the abstract. In Koestler, A., and Smythies, J. R. (Eds.): *Beyond Reductionism* (New York, Macmillan, 1969).

ceptual structures of a model representation. Items have an unbounded number of properties. We "see" them in terms of those properties of interest and concern to us. We construe items in a particular way, that is, we *achieve* interpretations by assigning conceptual structures to signs. In seeing that an object X is of a certain kind, as cognitive agents, we also can infer that Y follows as a consequence. There are real patterns out there in the world, but our knowledge of them, truth$_2$ contains an element of interpretation that derives from us as not only a type of complex and capricious organism but also from our presuppositions and background assumptions as types of persons living in social communities. We are cognitive agents with higher-order capacities, able to construct new beliefs (i.e. going beyond the simple receiving of information signs).

Inquirer: I can't easily accept that it is so much a matter of interpretation. Humans can conceive of so many possible interpretations, we would never reach an agreement. In your sketch of Figure 2, different interpreters may have different conceptual nets depending on their anatomies, endocrines, and personal histories. They may construe or classify signs in widely different ways. What happens to objectivity under this interpretational view?

Metaphysician: There may be an indefinite number of conceptually possible interpretations, but there also exist a large number of internal as well as external constraints that drastically narrow the viable and workable candidates. Remember, there are real lawful objective patterns out there, and their own nature restricts our readings if we want these readings to be accurate enough to interact with these patterns successfully. Laws constrain the range of states an object can exhibit in a domain. Our interpretations are products of the mind *but not of the mind alone*. The object has a say-so in the types of signs emanating from it as a source.

You and I both agree that the object is an apple. We might disagree about it being a delicious apple. But neither of us will construe the apple as an elephant or an orchid. Interpretations of informational signs by humans are not as unbounded and arbitrary as you seem to fear. General principles are involved, but there is also room for individual idiosyncrasy. By step-wise resolutions, we can progressively reduce personal subjective elements deriving from, and sensitive to, personal histories. We can calibrate and make adjustments for idiosyncrasy, as the history of science shows. Objectivity, or, if you wish, "semi-objectivity," is a consequence of agreed-on intersubjective testability; it is centered around equivalent human observers achieving similar interpretations because they themselves are so similar, having much in common.

Inquirer: Why would you and I agree on anything? I suppose we can be viewed as copies or repetitions of *Homo sapiens*. We are similarly constructed biologically, we receive similar physical wave forms that modulate the activity of similar nervous systems, we have been brought up in similar cultures, and we share the same language as well as a large number of beliefs and presuppositions. A child, a housewife, a farmer, and a botanist might have differently elaborated conceptual structures for an apple based on their interests and beliefs, but at some level of commonality they would agree the object in question is an apple. Isn't there something that is the "essence" of an apple?

Metaphysician: The ancient notion that objects have an essence, a fixed set of necessary and sufficient defining properties, is currently being revived and discussed by philosophers.[21] The trouble with

[21]See Kripke, S.: *Naming and Necessity* (Cambridge, Harvard University Press, 1980), as well as Putnam, H.: *Philosophical Papers, Vol. II: Mind Language and Reality* (Cambridge, Cambridge
→

essentialism in science is that scientists keep redescribing and redefining their objects. We never have the last word. What is taken as fundamental by one generation is taken as derivative by the next. The atomic number of gold — 79 — may currently now be considered its essence. But what will a future physics say about some property or properties more fundamental than atomic number?

Inquirer: I can see how, at least for a time being, we can agree on what is gold and what are apples. They are concrete, physical things. Human actions are so complex, it is hard to see how we will come to agree on our interpretations of them.

Metaphysician: Complexity is not an argument against agreement. Complexity is a methodological, not an ontological, category. Everything is complex. To you, a drop of water is not complex, but to a modern physical chemist, it still remains very mysterious. Physicists get good agreements on their interpretations in part because they deal with simple quantifiable properties such as space, time, and number. They can correlate their interpretations with quantitative perceptual pointer-readings that everyone can agree on. They have not only a theoretical structure and an empirical structure but also epistemic correlations or correspondence rules that relate the two.

Take the history of the concept of temperature.[22] At first it began with the purely qualitative notion that two bodies had the same temperature if, to our organs for heat sensation, one was not experienced as hotter than another or no change in hotness of either body was noticed when the bodies were brought together. Then a

---

[22]The following account is taken from the superb Lenzen, V. F.: *The Nature of Physical Theory* (New York, John Wiley, 1931).

University Press, 1979). For a rebuttal, see Shapere, D.: Reason, reference and the quest of knowledge (*Philosophy of Science, 49*:1, 1982), as well as Fales, E.: Natural kinds and freaks of nature (*Philosophy of Science, 49*:67, 1982).

correlation was noted in that as a body became heated, its volume increased. This correlation was indeed a lucky one for us because we can measure volume quantitatively. Hence, thermometers were invented. Now we look at the length of a column of mercury in a scaled glass tube. We have a pointer reading we can agree on. We agree the top of the column is lined up at, say, 98.6. But notice that this pointer reading, to be useful, must be interpreted or construed as representing the concept of temperature. Any small child could tell you the top of the red line in the tube is at a line with a number on it. But he does not know the significance of this match. You have to have a certain background knowledge to know what a reading of 98.6 means. It looks simple to us now, but it took bright people several hundred years to work this all out.

When the concepts involve complex human actions, things are not so easy because the human sciences are still in the fledgling stage. But let's try to get them off the ground. As realists, we will assume there is an order to an independent world and we can acquire knowledge as to its patterns, making it intelligible *for us* as a species. We assume that there exist individual humans with properties. We group individuals into classes based on clusters of properties. Some of these properties can be associated in the law-like relations (i.e. regular associations between two or more properties). Remember laws and rules apply to our models of the world, which are always limited, since they are based on current knowledge. But to get started you have to first find properties to define the classes of kinds which come to be used as terms in the laws. If a law statement asserts "all metals are conductors," there must be agreement on the nature of the kinds "metals" and "conductors." Before you get

	to the law stage, you have to work through the "what is it?" stage. To say what something is involves construing it in a particular way (i.e. the "which" of William James). In short, you need a preliminary classification of kinds. These kinds form the basis necessary for inductive generalizations.[23]
Inquirer:	The "what is it?" we consider to be a crisis problem of current psychiatry. But many psychiatrists simply don't see it as a crisis or predicament or even as a quandary. They complacently think it will all be worked out in time under the current DSM-III system. They don't see its unreliabilities as examples of the system being unworkable in that we don't know what we are dealing with. What *is* it we are dealing with?
Metaphysician:	That sounds like a scientific question beyond my scope. Before you can get to the *why, how,* or *how come*, you have to decide on the *what* and *which*. I do not know exactly what it is you are dealing with. You say you are dealing with mental disorders which sounds to me like you are dealing with abnormal internal models, skewed conceptual construals in certain people. All I can say is that realism and pragmatism would seem to be the effective world views for your purposes in psychiatry as long as you understand these are extra-scientific metaphysical beliefs.[24] You do not

---

[23]The history of psychiatry, psychology, and many of the behavioral sciences has been that they have been trying to run too quickly before they even learned to crawl, perhaps driven by the urge to earn the cachet of respectability called "science" exemplified by physics and chemistry. But these fields first had to agree on distinct kinds, such as "water," "ice," "glass," "mineral," etc., in which each kind exhibits certain clusters or concatenations of traits taken as fixed for the time being. See Nagel, E.: *The Structure of Science* (New York, Harcourt Brace and World, 1961). "The discovery and classification of kinds is an early but indispensable stage in the development of systematic knowledge, and all the sciences, including physics and chemistry, assume as well as continue to refine and modify distinctions with respect to kinds that have been initially recognized in common experience. Indeed, the development of comprehensive theoretical systems seems to be possible *only after a preliminary classification of kinds has been achieved*" (italics added), p. 31.

[24]We might also keep in mind Einstein's remarks on epistemological opportunism quoted earlier.

want to just experience or enjoy or be in harmony with the world. You want dependable, interventionist knowledge to change the world. You want to become more efficacious in intervening in order to rid it of some of its humanly undesirable properties and to be able to preserve what is humanly worthwhile. Max Frisch remarked that technology was the knack of so arranging the world that we do not have to experience it.[25] A pragmatic realism will provide you with the most fruitful metaphysical blueprint for your purposes. You will have to consult scientists about the *what* of your problem domain.

Inquirer: Scientists are therefore next on my list. I thank you for such a profound and enlightening excursion, not often heard in the narrow corridors of psychiatric argumentation.

---

[25]See Frisch, M.: *Homo Faber.*

THE BIOLOGICAL SCIENTIST

THE Inquirer consults the Biological Scientist. She is not a molecular biologist. She is well versed in the problems of taxonomy and theoretical biology. She looks astute and a bit wary of what this is all about.

Inquirer: Psychiatry is concerned with the etiology, diagnosis, prognosis, treatment and prevention of mental disorders. Let's put aside the rest of this nest of nettles and attend only to the core question of diagnosis.

Biological
Scientist: What do you mean by diagnosis in psychiatry?

Inquirer: The term comes from medicine. To make a diagnosis is to classify a patient according to the disease or diseases he possesses. We convert input evidence into an output of names of diseases which are conceptual entities that identify or explain abnormalities in the evidence.[1]

Biological
Scientist: More precisely, diagnosis seems not to be classification but identification. You identify the patient as belonging to one or more disease classes or categories that have been established by someone else who had developed the classification scheme.

Inquirer: I accept the refinement. We identify or recognize patients as members of classes of disorders.

Biological
Scientist: How do you decide whether an individual patient belongs in a given class?

Inquirer: By a combination of demographic and clinical properties the patient manifests. The clinical properties are signs and symptoms gathered from a history and examination of the patient supplemented by numerous laboratory tests.

---

[1]See Feinstein, A. R.: An analysis of diagnostic reasoning, 1973, p. 212.

Biological
Scientist: Offhand, the procedure appears sound enough to me.
               What is the difficulty you are having in psychiatry?

Inquirer: The difficulty lies in a lack of agreement among the
               psychiatrists as to which category the patient belongs.
               Judges show poor rates of agreement for most
               diagnostic categories. Thus the categories are unreliable
               in the everyday sense of the term. One would not con-
               sider them to represent dependable knowledge.

Biological
Scientist: Are the categories too vaguely defined or are the criteria
               of application lacking?

Inquirer: What is the difference from your viewpoint?

Biological
Scientist: A definition consists of terms which designate the mean-
               ing of a class-concept by describing the properties
               shared by members of the class. The terms used should
               not be too vague. Vagueness implies it is difficult to
               determine what limits the user of a term intended to put
               on its inclusiveness, making the boundaries of the class
               term unclear. The term *patriotic* designates a vague class
               because it is extremely difficult to specify its meaning
               and therefore who is and who is not patriotic. A
               criterion is a test to be applied that tells you whether an
               individual possesses the properties stated in the defini-
               tion. For example, a chemist may define copper as the
               element having an atomic number of 29. But this defini-
               tion does not at all help you decide whether the lump of
               metal you have in hand is made of copper. You would
               have to test it for malleability, electrical conductivity,
               melting point (1083° C), etc. to determine if the lump is
               an instance of copper. Litmus paper can tell you if a liq-
               uid is an acid, but the litmus paper test does not tell you
               what it means to be an acid.

Inquirer: I suppose in psychiatry we suffer both from vague
               definitions and a lack of criterial tests for forming a
               reliable classification.

Biological
Scientist: Classifications are difficult. Here is one that you might

want to add to your collection. A ninth century Chinese encyclopedia, called the *Celestial Emporium of Benevolent Knowledge*, divided animals into the following classes:

a. Those that belong to the Emperor
b. Embalmed ones
c. Those that are trained
d. Suckling pigs
e. Mermaids
f. Fabulous ones
g. Stray dogs
h. Those that are included in this classification
i. Those that tremble as if they were mad
j. Innumerable ones
k. Those drawn with a very fine camel's hair brush.
l. Others
m. Those that have just broken the flower vase
n. Those that resemble flies from a distance.[2]

I like the group "others" because Linnaeus, the father of classification in modern biology, also had a class he couldn't fit organisms into easily. He called it "chaos."

Inquirer: I like item (h). It illustrates the humor of self-reference which has many parallels in mathematics, music and art.[3] But I digress. How could we go about improving our situation?

Biological
Scientist: I don't know, but I can give you some examples from biological taxonomy.

Inquirer: Please elucidate.

Biological
Scientist: Let me re-emphasize what the Metaphysician told you in his philosophic way. A taxonomy involves kinds, and kinds are in part cognitive instruments fashioned to

---

[2]The fabled classification is from an essay by Borges, "The Analytical Language of John Wilkins."

[3]See Hofstadter, *Gödel, Escher, Bach*, p. 495, Heady thoughts about self-reference can be very mind-bending. See Goodman, N.: *Languages of Art: An Approach To A Theory of Symbols* (New York, Bobbs-Merrill, 1968, p. 59). "A symbol that denotes itself also exemplifies itself, is both denoted and exemplified by itself. 'Word' is thus related to itself, and so are 'short' and 'polysyllabic,' but not 'long' or 'monosyllabic.' 'Long' is a sample of 'short,' 'monosyllabic' denotes short words, and 'short' both exemplifies and denotes short words."

serve human purposes. In biology, in forming "natural" kinds, we select characters or properties of living things depending on our interests and concerns. The question is whether the kinds we fashion conform satisfactorily to the order or pattern or natural kinds existing in the real world. One trouble you might be having in psychiatry is that the known disease signs and symptoms represent too few properties for a reliable classification. That is, there are undiscovered pieces to the puzzle missing. Or perhaps you do not have the right properties to begin with.

Inquirer: What do you mean by "right"?

Biological
Scientist: To quote our taxonomic forefather, Linnaeus, the first step in science is to know one thing from another. Let's say we start with a collection of individuals of some sort — organisms, specimens, people, patients — that we are going to delimit into subgroups. We know that no two individuals are completely identical. Living organisms show great diversity and idiosyncrasy but that does not mean they are not comparable. At the simplest level we might say, using a class concept, that individuals are similar in that they share a character, a quality, a property. If they share a single property, they are members of a class (e.g. all red things). If they share a set of properties, they constitute a kind, (e.g. *Homo sapiens*). If the properties can be lawfully related, we have what I call a "natural" kind. In biological taxonomy we have tried to construct natural kinds, taxa whose members are tolerably alike. The right properties are those that lead to a natural kind, a taxon, in which there is a high information content about members of the kind. [4]

Inquirer: In biology, how do you use what you term a "taxon"

---

[4]It is not quite as clear-cut as the Biological Scientist is making it out to be. Perhaps she has expository purposes. The concept of species as a natural kind works well with animals but not so well with plants. A "natural kind" may imply to the unreflective that exactly that kind really exists in nature independent of ourselves and all we have to do is find it. It further implies "essentialism," the doctrine that some properties are essential to an object, whereas others are not. This view overlooks the contribution we ourselves as observers and as species make in choosing and interpreting signs as characteristic of an object. Many characteristics of an object lie beyond our senses because our capacity to receive signs is limited. That organisms emit infrared radiation was unknown until relatively recently
→

Biological
Scientist:

with high information content?

Knowing an individual is a member of a kind, one can make many inferences about his additional properties without going through all the trouble of examining him further to ascertain them. One can make predictions about the individual. It is certainly useful to anticipate what you can expect in the future when you try to navigate through the world. A classification scheme serves as a convenient information storage and retrieval system.

In biology, there is another purpose to a taxonomy besides discovering or constructing an order in living systems. Species serve not only as a unit of classification but also as a unit of evolution. We believe the taxa or kinds somehow reflect the process of evolution which brought about a great diversity of organisms. Whatever caused evolution caused this particular order or arrangement of organisms into taxa.[5] Thus far, evolutionary biologists believe that the combined operation of random

---

because we cannot directly perceive these wavelengths. We must infer their existence through long lines of inference and reasoning. There must be many more as yet undiscovered characteristics in our world. So, what may be considered essential now might not hold in the future. It has been doubted there exist totally independent natural kinds because any pair of non-identical objects share an equal number of properties as any other pair when the number of properties is finite. See Watanabe's "theorem of the ugly duckling." In Watanabe, S.: *Knowing and Guessing* (New York, John Wiley, 1969, p. 376). Hence, to form a kind, properties must be selected and weighted.

A new technology revealing new properties can revise a classification because a new spectrum of individuals is now involved. Who are we to say what is an "essential" property? It may be only essential to us, at a particular time and for particular purposes. We might use the term *natural kind* to mean that the kind is in accord both with what is out there and with ourselves as part of nature. The whole issue of a natural kind is quite controversial and spiritedly debated by philosophers of science as well as by biologists. Before Darwin, the British philosopher Whewell (pronounced for mysterious reasons "Hew-well") stated: "The maxim by which all sytems professing to be natural must be tested is this: that the arrangement obtained from one set of characters coincides with the arrangement obtained from another." See Whewell, W.: *Philosophy of Inductive Science* (London, John Parker, 1847). Cf. also Simpson, *Principles of Animal Taxonomy.* Also, see Pratt, Y. S. F.: Biological classification (*British Journal for the Philosophy of Science, 23*:305, 1972), and Mellor, D. H.: Natural kinds (*British Journal for the Philosophy of Science, 28*:299, 1977), as well as Levin D. A.: The nature of plant species (*Science, 204*:381, 1979).

[5] Thus, biology has three competing taxonomic systems involving similarity of organisms by possession of shared properties, by possession of a common ancestor, and by a combination of genealogy and degree of divergence. Each system gives somewhat different clusterings. Using outward appearances, who would guess that birds and crocodiles have a common ancestor? See Mayr, E.: Biological classifications: toward a synthesis of opposing methodologies (*Science, 214*:510, 1981), as well as his massive historical survey, *Growth of Biological Thought: Diversity Evolution and Inheritance* (Cambridge, Belknap, 1982, p. 147).

variation and natural selection is the causal mechanism. "Random" in this context does not mean mathematically random in the sense of equally likely, but only that the variations are "blind" and do not arise because they preferentially lead to anticipated and advantageous traits.[6]

But there are undoubtedly additional mechanisms at work as well in evolution. In psychiatry, if you found a group of patients sharing the same disorder, wouldn't you tend to believe the causal mechanisms involved are the same?

Inquirer: Perhaps, but causality in the domain of disorders can be quite complex. Cause A can produce related effects B1 and B2; A can have unrelated effects B1 or B2; B1 or B2 can lead to the same effect C; A can cause B which causes C (that is, without A, C will not occur); the conjoint A1 and A2 can cause B, and so forth.[7] Even when you know causes, the "why," it does not provide an understanding of the intervening processes, the "what" is going on. The "why" may be long gone, and what you have left to intervene in is the "what." The blow on the head happened yesterday and now you are dealing with internal bleeding in the brain.

We are far away from determining causes in most of psychiatry. First, we must be able to classify and identify people with disorders. No doubt biology has been able to develop an increasingly reliable taxonomy. What is the secret of this success?

Biological
Scientist: The non-secret is hard work over a long period of time.

---

[6]Note 16 in Dialogue IV introduced the concept of randomness as referring not to a haphazard lack of structure but to a structure with a probabilistic element in it. This element is a random variable that can assume any one of a set of values in accordance with the operation of some probabilistic, stochastic process. A random number is one in which, in the sequence of integers, each integer is independent of one another, one having no bearing on the occurrence of another in the sequence. The entire sequence, however, is generated systematically by a random number generator that follows rules. Thus, a random number sequence is not disordered. Its order can represent the decimal expansion of a fraction, in fact an infinity of fractions. The biological concept of the randomness is akin to this mathematical concept in their sharing of a notion of independence. Random genetic change is not a result of "sizing up" the environment and producing an advantageous variation. Genetic changes are "blind" to their ultimate effects on the organism and to offspring.

[7]Cause-effect relations are taken up again in Dialogue VII with "The Clinical Psychologist," and their further complexities are elaborated in Dialogue VIII with "The Psychiatric Scientist."

A lot of dedicated people have worked on the problem of constructing a "natural" classification. In a sense, all classifications are non-natural or artificial in that they represent human constructions and there are indefinitely many constructions that can be formed. The term *natural* no longer means to me that the classes exist in nature exactly as we conceived them, but that they are good and useful approximations to an order out there. Perhaps the term *relevant kind* would be better than *natural kind* and we could speak of weak and strong relevance. If you use incidental or accidental properties, you form a classification with low information content, like the phone books' alphabetical ordering of people's names. Such a weak relevant kind consists, for example, of the people whose last name begins with the letter A. The kind is useful for the single purpose of finding a person's phone number and address, but it's not rich enough in information content to comprise a taxon whose members share many properties. Biologists started with the manifest properties of overall morphological similarities between organisms. They then ordered the organisms according to these similarities.

Inquirer: At the start, how did they pick the organisms for the initial collection?

Biological
Scientist: By simple visual inspection of outward appearances and using common sense. It is obvious to our pattern-recognizing abilities of manifest properties that some specimens of organisms are more alike in shape than others. Perceptual judgments are quickly settled interpretations. Plants differ from animals, and dogs are more like cats than like monkeys. The basic idea is to arrange or order the initial collection into groups based on resemblances. At the start, you may be including atypical cases and excluding cases which should be in the group. If you cluster individuals in an initial collection that you think are animals, and one or two eventually turns out to be extremely distant in resemblance to the others, it's no great loss. Outward appearances were the starting point, but they are not enough. In the insect world, the male and female of the species may not

look at all alike. Or consider the caterpillar and the butterfly. A sea anemone looks like a plant but it is an animal.

A taxon whose members resemble one another in many ways will have a high information content for the purpose of the classification. Knowing an individual is a member of a strong relevant kind, one can automatically derive a large number of predictions about him. In time, the members of this kind will be discovered to share many new properties in addition to those used initially to construct the classification. These new properties may not be manifest to simple inspection. They may be underlying properties at a deeper level. For example, man was grouped with chimpanzee by the nineteenth century taxonomists on grounds of gross morphological similarities. With the advent of the use of chemical properties in the 1960s, it was found that man and chimpanzee shared 99 percent of their structural genes. As I said, knowing that an individual is a member of a reliable taxon allows you to make a large number of correct inferences about him. Cognitively, this is very satisfying and expedient, providing a great economy of thought. It allows you to anticipate events you might not otherwise foresee. It is hard to predict, especially the future.

Inquirer: The first step in biology was finding the properties in a starting collection and then estimating the resemblances between individuals with those properties.

Biological
Scientist: Right. Properties are associated in clusters. In biology, there are roughly two sorts of clusters of kinds, monothetic and polythetic.[8] A monothetic kind is one in which each member must possess all the properties used in defining the kind. Unless an individual possesses properties A + B + C + D, he is excluded from the kind. In psychiatry, when you define a schizophrenic as being under age thirty *and* unmarried *and* having delusions *and* having hallucinations, you are offering an ex-

---

[8]The formulation comes from Beckner, M.: *The Biological Way of Thought* (New York, Columbia University Press, 1959) and the terms from Sneath, P. H. A., and Sokal, R.: *Numerical Taxonomy* (San Francisco, W. H. Freeman, 1973). The latter is a rugged in-depth tome covering all aspects of taxonomy.

ample of a monothetic kind. A polythetic kind is much looser. Each member need possess only a large number of the kind-defining properties, each property is possessed by large numbers of the individuals, and no property is necessarily possessed by every member of the kind. A kind is polythetic if the first two conditions are fulfilled and fully polythetic if all three are satisfied.[9]

Inquirer: When you have only one or two properties shared by members of a kind, the degree of resemblance is weak. A strong natural kind is one in which the individuals share many properties of different sorts.

Biological
Scientist: A maximally strong natural kind would be a group which shared several laws. Scientists look for laws as properties, objective patterns of generalization. Kinds are first needed to serve as bound variables in these generalizations. A law-like statement describes a regularity as an objective pattern. It states this is the way the real world is hooked together, the way things happen.[10]

Inquirer: A maximally strong natural kind, or taxon, would be a group based on its laws. Laws restrict the possible states and changes of states in individuals in a class. Maybe there are no laws which characterize psychiatric patients.

Biological
Scientist: There must be laws or principles at some level,

---

[9]A few questions are being begged here. What is a large number? (A large number is one whose logarithm is a large number). In spite of some difficulties with this distinction between monothetic and polythetic kinds, it will be useful for psychiatric taxonomy because it constantly reminds us of the logic involved in forming clusters. When we attribute a property to an individual, we perform a cognitive act because we are actually assigning an attribute or predicate to our representation or model of that individual. Model representations are conceptual sketches and do not cover every detail. We believe that there is some sort of correspondence between the property we assign in our internal models and the property the real individual has. There are purely conceptual properties that we can assign to an individual, knowing they do not represent a real substantive property but are simply reflections of an attribute in the model we ascribe for our own purposes. For example, the metal gold possesses mass as a substantive property. We as persons attribute a high price to gold. In a chemical context, we would consider the price of gold to be incidental, but not so in a financial context.
[10]Again, the Biological Scientist offers idealizations, which is what laws and theories are. Biological laws are not strict, exceptionless generalizations like many of those that have been proposed in classical mechanics. It is a law in biology that vertebrates possess red blood cells. But ice fish have been discovered that have no red blood cells.
→

otherwise the world is not ordered and successful science would not be possible the way it has been. Perhaps you have not yet formulated law-like statements that apply to your current model of your domain. The laws may be extremely elusive, probabilistic or complex, but they are potentially describable as statements about objective patterns. I would think you need to know laws, generalizations, principles, or at least rough rules if you are going to treat similar patients in similar ways. Wouldn't it be a useful rule that stated if you give treatment X to patients of class Y, the outcome will be Z with some likelihood? You could have a special-purpose classification that not all scientists might not find useful. You might even base a classification on treatment response.

Inquirer: At the moment we have only the course of an illness and treatment response as prediction criteria. But what is the treatment being applied to? Could one treat a patient on a particular dimension without saying he is a member of a kind?

Biological
Scientist: A dimension is a single characteristic or property. It represents a class, albeit weak in information content compared to a taxon. But one dimension might be all the information you need for clinical purposes. If you looked at patients along a number of dimensions, you could form stronger groups by clustering the patients according to their values on these dimensions. Because forming kinds is a conceptual act, you can group any collection of individuals into clusters. But will the clusters be applicatively useful?

Inquirer: This seems to be simple pragmatism. I thought scientists tried to understand and appreciate the way the world works. They supposedly take intellectual pleasure in searching for truth for its own sake independent of

---

Now what should we do? Should we say these fish are invertebrates or say the law holds probabilistically most of the time and absorb the anomaly? As another example, the presence of enucleated erythrocytes would group mammals with some salamanders. Toleration of anomalous exceptions for the time being is necessary, as the history of science has repeatedly shown. There is no single measure of similarity. The pragmatic course is not to rely on single properties but to order clusters of diversity in a multidimensional character space.

vulgar pragmatic concerns.

Biological
Scientist: There is no nutshell definition of science. Science satisfies a wide range of cognitive and pragmatic interests. There are all kinds of scientists, many of whom, particularly theoreticians, would endorse your last statement. But notice that if a theory is to be accepted as "true," the conceptual entities of the theory and their relations must somehow map onto the real entities and relations of the world. The clearest example is a theory that makes a prediction about the value of an observable property. When observation confirms the prediction at some approximation, we say the theory is correct or reliable in application.[11]

Inquirer: Classifications are not true or false either. As you and the Metaphysician have described them, they are artifacts constructed as cognitive tools for human purposes. Is a hammer or shoe true? A classification is justified, but isn't it strange to call it "true"?

Biological
Scientist: Yes, but a classification is an indispensable step towards correct theories that in the jargon we call "true." It is a matter of aptness and fit rather than truth.

---

[11]This is mainly because we have come to trust our methods of observation. The theory is not true because it works; it works because it is true (i.e. it fits the world well). The view is that of methodological pragmatism. Pure cognitive comfort or intellectual satisfaction can be strengthened by pragmatic success. Cf. Rescher, N., *Methodological Pragmatism*. Working scientists use the term *true* in a particular way as was pointed out in Dialogue IV. Except for dogmatists, they do not mean "This is the way it really is for all time."

The classical definition of truth was *Veritas est adaequatio rei et intellectus*. Sometimes this is translated as a "correspondence" between things and the mind. But correspondence requires that objects be similar. Two statements can correspond, as in Tarski's " 'Snow is white' is true if and only if snow is white," in which terms of the statement in the meta-language in single quotes have a correspondence with the last three terms of the statement in the object language. Philosophers take the Tarskian example as an issue of truth. For scientists, the factual question involves the natural language statement regarding empirical whiteness as a property of snow. The relation between the empirical fact and the statement is one of an *adaequatio* of description. "True" statements effectively describe (i.e. if they are followed as instructions, they get you where you want to go). Truer statements are more effective descriptions resulting in a greater efficacy of rational action. The relation is one of accommodation, a rough but successful key-and-lock fit between organism and environment. Nietzsche (of all people) described this sort of truth as "the kind of error without which a certain species of life could not live." See Nietzsche, F.: *The Will to Power*. Kaufman, W. (Ed.). (New York, Random House, 1967, p. 272).

→

You might think it strange to say that a hammer is true. But a shoe is a closer analogy. It fits or accommodates a foot to some degree of approximation. A shoe is fashioned more like a theory. It fits because it produces desired results in some context. Then we say it is provisionally true. A good classification is effective as an informational tool in our progressively stepwise aim of obtaining what we want to know truly.

Inquirer: It is obvious that psychiatry as a technology must have mainly pragmatic interventionist aims. However, pragmatic treatment aims in principle should be helped by knowledge gained through purely cognitive aims. A technology should be principled to be intelligible. Medicine advanced rapidly when its underlying sciences went beyond purely manifest properties and gained new knowledge at deeper levels. If we are to do better with psychiatric patients, we must know more about what kinds of patients they are. We do not have enough properties yet or enough of the underlying lawful properties to form a dependable classification scheme. In short, to find new groups we need new methods to get new evidence, new data, and new manifestations of disorder, which may reveal a new disorder or help separate currently overlapping disorders.

Biological
Scientist: To get new methods for assessing new properties, you first need new ideas. Also, you want to try to get different sets of properties. This allows you to maximize the number of inferences about the kind you are interested in. When a new technique indicating a new property is introduced, it is tried on members of a previously established kind. If the members of the

---

Incidentally, a will to power is the wish to have the power to satisfy all wishes. When asked the three-wishes questions, a smart child realizes he needs only one. It is hard to resist here another remark of Nietzsche's about truth: "What therefore is truth? A mobile army of metaphors, metonymies, anthropomorphisms; in short, a sum of human relaions which become rhetorically intensified, metamorphored, adorned, and after a long usage seem to a nation fixed, canonic, and binding; truths are illusions of which one has forgotten that they *are* illusions" (*On Truths and Lie in an Extramoral Sense*) in Kaufman, W. (Ed.), *The Portable Nietzsche*, (New York, Random House, 1954, p. 47).

group are found to also share the new property, then one gains confidence that this is a stable, relevant kind.

The success of modern biological taxonomy lies not in just having lots of properties but properties of different sorts at different levels. For example, in classifying animals we use morphological, physiological, biochemical, ecological and behavioral properties. It is the mutually corroborating convergence of these different sorts of properties that tightens up the affinity relations among members of a taxon and among different taxa. By "corroborating convergence," I mean a concatenation of evidence — a body of facts, interpretations, hypotheses, assumptions, inferences and lines of reasoning. This massive concatenation of evidence, which involves far more than empirical observation, builds up into a compelling argument. As a marvelous example, let me read to you a passage from the first chapter of Darwin's *Origin of Species*, a book which he called "one long argument." Darwin is discussing the hypothesis that all breeds of domestic pigeons have a common origin in the rock pigeon.

If the several breeds are not varieties, and have not proceeded from the rock pigeon, they must have descended from at least seven or eight aboriginal stocks; for it is impossible to make the present domestic breeds by the crossing of any lesser number. . . . The supposed aboriginal stocks must all have been rock pigeons, that is, they did not breed or willingly perch on trees. But besides *C. livia*, with its geographical sub-species, only two or three other species of rock pigeon are known; and these have not any of the characters of the domestic breeds. Hence the supposed aboriginal stocks must either still exist in the countries where they were originally domesticated, and yet be unknown to ornithologists; and this, considering their size, habits, and remarkable characters, seems improbable; or they must have become extinct in the wild state. But birds breeding on precipices, and good fliers, are unlikely to be exterminated; and the common rock pigeon, which has the same habits with the domestic breeds, has not been exterminated even on several of the smaller British islets, or on the shores of the Mediterranean. Hence the supposed extermination of so many species having similar habits with the rock pigeon seems a very rash assumption. Moreover, the several above-named domesticated breeds have been transported to all parts of the world, and, therefore, some of them must have been carried back again into their native country; but not one has become wild or feral. . . . Again, all recent experience shows that it is difficult to get wild animals to breed freely under domestication; yet, on the hypothesis of the multiple origin of our pigeons, it must be assumed that at least seven or eight species were so thoroughly domesticated in ancient times by half-civilized man, as to be quite prolific under confinement. The above-specified breeds, though agreeing generally with the wild rock pigeon in constitution, habits, voice, coloring, and in most parts of their structure, yet are certainly highly abnormal in other parts. . . . Hence it must be assumed not only that half-civilized man succeeded in thoroughly domesticating abnormal species; and further, that these very species have since all become extinct or unknown. So many strange contingencies are improbable in the highest degree.

Some facts in regard to the coloring of pigeons well deserve consideration. . . . We can understand these facts, on the well-known principle of reversion to ancestral characters, if all the domestic breeds are descended from the rock pigeon. But if we deny this, we must make one of the two following highly improbable suppositions. Either, first, that all the several imagined aboriginal stocks were colored and marked like the rock pigeon, although no other existing species is thus colored and marked, so that in each separate breed there might be a tendency to revert to the very same colors and markings. Or, secondly, that each breed, even the purest, has within a dozen, or at most within a score, of generations, been crossed by the rock pigeon. . . .

Lastly, the hybrids or mongrels from between all the breeds of the pigeon are perfectly fertile, as I can state from my own observations, purposely made, on the most distinct breeds. Now, hardly any cases have been ascertained with certainty of hybrids from two quite distinct species of animals being perfectly fertile. . . .

From these several reasons, namely, the improbability of man having formerly made seven or eight supposed species of pigeons to breed freely under domestication: these supposed species being quite unknown in a wild state, and their not having become anywhere feral; these species presenting certain very abnormal characters, as compared with all other *Columbidae*, though so like the rock pigeon in most respects; the occasional re-appearance of the blue color and various black marks in all the breeds, both when kept pure and when crossed; and lastly, the mongrel offspring being perfectly fertile; from these several reasons taken together, we may safely conclude that all our domestic breeds are descended from the rock pigeon or *Columa livia* with its geographical sub-species.[12]

Inquirer: Now that is what I would call a compelling argument! If the entire book is one long argument, it must be very long indeed. Your quotation is long enough.[13] Notice

---

[12]See Darwin, C.: *Origin of Species* (London, John Murray, 1859).

[13]The book you are now reading is also one very long argument. In complex problems, long thoughts are needed.

how he wove together a large number of kinds of evidence to build and buttress his position.

Biological
Scientist: I would think it is this sort of body of evidence — facts, inferences, theories, interpretations, all pieced together — that you need in psychiatry. I am a biological scientist. Why don't you talk with behavioral scientists like psychologists?

Inquirer: Coming up.

Dialogue VI

THE MIND SCIENTIST

T HE Mind Scientist is a new breed of cat on the scene, a
psychologist having one foot in cognitive psychology and the
other in artificial intelligence. His domain is now called the
"cognitive sciences." His ultimate aim is to explain human mental
processes using computational concepts, theories, models and
methods.

Inquirer: It has long been argued that there exists a fundamental
difference between the natural sciences, such as physics
and chemistry, and those sciences which attempt to explain human behavior. Some even claim there can be
no science of human behavior because of the inherent
variability and idiosyncrasy of human individuals.

Mind
Scientist: This is a version of the ancient "similar-different" con-
undrum. When are two things the same? A profound
question.[1] If they are exactly the same in all respects,
then you have only one thing. What is a "one" and what
is a "two"? No two objects are alike in all respects, and
all objects are alike in some respects. Our problem is
how to best organize this observed diversity. When
nineteenth century philosophers made the distinction
between *Naturwissenschaften* and *Geisteswissenschaften*, the
latter being a branch of the humanities, they were not
only drawing attention to two kinds of objects of
knowledge, one of nature and one of human minds, but
also to differences in methods for obtaining these
knowledges.[2]

---

[1]For a thoroughgoing contemporary treatment of the issues involved, see Wiggins, D.:
Sameness and Substance (Cambridge, Harvard University Press, 1980).
[2]It seems strange to us, now pursuing the last fifth of the twentieth century, that mental processes were then not viewed as "natural" or part of nature. Perhaps there was confusion regarding those aspects of mental processes biologically inherited and those aspects acquired

→

81

The methods of the natural sciences, like physics and chemistry, were cognitively satisfying and pragmatically successful in managing the problems of their subject matter. But when applied to problems of mental activity, these methods might not be so successful or even appropriate. I must admit they had a point because twentieth century behavioral sciences, such as psychology and sociology, have not been exactly spectacular in their achievements despite the availability of all sorts of sophisticated statistical, survey, and experimental paraphernalia.[3] Maybe we have not yet found the right methodology. I still believe a science of mental activity is eventually possible because, as the Metaphysician indicated, mental processes, as part of the natural order, are ordered and lawful at some level. The social or human sciences are still at a largely programmatic stage. You must give us time and bright people. Promises, promises, but at least not threats, threats as you get from our institutions.

Inquirer: What is the big difference between the natural and mental sciences?

Mind
Scientist: First, let's consider a few general points about scientific fields.

---

through experience, especially with the socio-symbolic environment. The latter aspects are man-guided and man-perturbed. Hence, part of mental processes are artifacts, man-shaped conceptual objects. Artifact kinds, such as clocks, are characterized not by what they are made of but by what their functions are. Clocks function as timekeepers and they can be made out of all sorts of materials. That we qualify as both natural and artifact kinds makes many people uncomfortable because nowadays it relates us more closely to computers, which, in part, function like we do. There will be a great deal of talk about this disaffection as we proceed.

[3]Still the best introduction to the behavioral sciences and its methods is Kaplan, A.: *The Conduct of Inquiry: Methodology for Behavioral Science* (San Francisco, Chandler, 1964). It is especially valuable as an antidote to the stultifying hup-two-three schools of methodology "forever perfecting how to do something without ever getting around to doing it even imperfectly" (p. 25). Methodology really should mean the study of methods, but we are now stuck with it as referring to the methods themselves. The behavioral mental sciences are sciences in the same sense as the natural sciences, but not in the same way. As will be seen, they are sciences in the same sense in that they attempt to move from manifest patterns of phenomena to underlying generative structures that produce or are responsible for these patterns. See Bhaskar, R.: *The Possibility of Naturalism: A Philosophical Critique of the Contemporary Human Sciences* (New Jersey, Humanities Press, 1979).

A field has a paradigm or a research tradition it relies on.[4] The discipline recognizes and classifies its particular objects of inquiry, and it has a proprietary vocabulary for talking about those objects or entities that constitute its subject matter. It selects problems to solve, and it has ways of deciding what are acceptable solutions.[5] It has methodological do's and don'ts. It studies non-random patterns and regularities, attempting to form law-like generalizations. It offers theories and models that try to explain why the laws are as they are and not otherwise. And a scientific field has underlying world views, as the Metaphysician pointed out. The major issues between the natural and mental sciences have centered around problems of reduction, of intention, and of interpretation. Let's start with reduction but not spend too much time on it because it is nowadays something of a tiresome issue, at least for me.

Inquirer: What made it so tiresome to you?

Mind
Scientist: The arguments eventually became too crazy and undiscussible. People overlooked that levels, being constructs, are not really things and, hence, do not causally act on one another. The original idea was that we could conceive of a pyramid of levels of sciences with physics at the bottom and sociology, say, at the top.[6] Sociology could be "reduced" to psychology, psychology to biology, biology to chemistry and chemistry to physics. But the term *reduction* in this spatial metaphor turned out to have a lot of confounded meanings. Reduction might mean that A provides the basis for B, such as the brain for the mind. Or it might mean A explains B or that

---

[4]Kuhn started everyone talking about paradigms. See Kuhn, *Structure of Scientific Revolutions* (p. 43). Originally, *paradeigmia* meant "example" in the sense of an exemplar to which things could be compared to see if they were members of the class exemplified by the paradigmatic case. In a postscript to the second edition (1970), Kuhn prefers the more comprehensive term *disciplinary matrix* to *paradigm* (p. 182). The concept of a research tradition comes from Laudan, L.: *Progress and Its Problems* (Berkeley, University of California Press, 1977).

[5]As mentioned in the introduction of this book, Poincaré, a fine mathematician, remarked that even in mathematics there are no solved problems; there are only problems more or less solved. Cf. Klein, M., *Mathematics* (p. 316).

[6]A typical textbook diagram looks like Figure 3.

knowledge of A predicts the behavior of B.

Wildly rococo claims were made such as explaining the United Nations in terms of the laws of thermodynamics. Reductionism is often just a put-down, an idea that has curdled. Much of the dispute looked like pygmies in the rain forest fighting over territories and over who was better than whom. If one adopts this pyramid metaphor as a vantage point, one can imply a hierarchy of rank orders in which one science is "higher" or "better" than another if the relation between the above and the below is one of dominance. But it could be one of many relations, for example, precedence. A hierarchy is a useful relation, but to view all of scientific knowledge as a hierarchy is to inflate a local property into a global one and to invite invidious comparisons. A web or network with relations of enmeshment is a more suitable metaphor than one of the dominance and subordination of a pecking order.

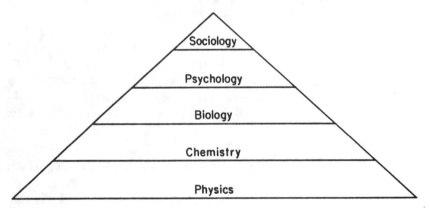

Figure 3. To move (conceptually) from the bottom to the top is to move from a level of more numerous objects to a level of less numerous objects. There are more electrons than human families. Or one could interpret it as a precedence ordering of historical time with the objects of physics at the beginning of the world and culminating with those of current sociology.

Inquirer: But isn't chemistry reducible to physics?
Mind
Scientist: Yes and no. Chemistry presupposes physics, but the reductions achieved did not make chemistry go away. Theories may be reducible, but not whole fields. Even in the pyramid metaphor, reductions connect and relate levels but do not abolish them. It is easy to confuse

reducibility with *applicability*. Physics and chemistry are not themselves objects but disciplines attending to conceived levels of organization of a world made up of objects. Levels are sets or classes and, therefore, they are human constructs. The levels are not static layers, because higher levels have been conceived to emerge over time from lower levels as the result of an evolutionary and development process. The higher levels are characterized by novel emergent properties not belonging to lower levels. Human organisms with particular mental processes comprise a new higher level. By "particular mental processes" I mean a set or network of powers to creatively manipulate symbols.

Inquirer: But aren't these powers a function of the central nervous system or brains of organisms? If so, why cannot mental processes be reduced to brain processes?

Mind
Scientist: I will grant that the ability to create and manipulate symbols in novel ways is supervenient on the brain and perhaps a few other ingredients, such as endocrines. If the symbolic processes of mentalling are a function or property of the brain, then they are not identical with the brain. An entity is not identical with one of its properties. The brain depends upon oxygen but it is not identical with oxygen. Water is composed of H_2O, but it has additional properties, such as transparency, that are not deducible from properties of atoms of hydrogen and oxygen alone. There is more to the *kind* water than its atomic constituents.

Inquirer: There are many thinkers who maintain that mental processes are identical with neural processes, the different terms being two ways of talking about one thing.[7] The temperature of a gas and the mean velocity of its molecules are taken as theoretically identical, as are genes and DNA molecules.

Mind
Scientist: Although phenomenologically they are quite distinct categorical domains, the mental and the neural can be related in several ways, identity being only one of them.

---

[7]See Wilson, E.: *The Mental as Physical* (London, Routledge and Kegan Paul, 1979).

A relation of theoretical identity can be drawn between heat and kinetic energy, mass and energy, and mind and brain, but the relation is interpretive (theoretical) and not observational. If you say the mental and the neural are identical, you must also say what they are identical *as*. Obviously, the mind and the brain are not identical objects, but their event structures might be identical. If so, a theoretical bridge law relating them would be in a bi-conditional form, stating that if A occurs in the mind, B occurs in the brain, and vice versa. The hard part is to specify under what descriptions mental-state kinds correlate with neural-state kinds.

Inquirer: Another way to relate the mental and neural would be to assert they are two manifestations of some other thing.

Mind
Scientist: Here we go again with what is a one and what is a two. If they are two manifestations, what is the third thing they are manifestations of? Davidson has proposed an anomalous (non-lawful) monism. He doubts there can be any strict psychophysical laws predicting and explaining mental phenomena because the mind-brain relations are only those between descriptions of correlated individual events and not between *kinds* of events.[8] Laws require specifications of kinds.

Inquirer: The brain's atomic constituents, at least for neuroscientists, are neurons. If mental activity is a function of the brain, how do you account for mental activity in terms of neurons?

Mind
Scientist: It is a claim of coarse resolving power to declare neurons are involved in mental processes. Studies of single neurons are not going to tell us much about what we want to know. Are you familiar with the Camel cigarette ad on Times Square in New York?

Inquirer: I am. The sign is a flashing billboard showing moving figures and printing funny comments.

Mind
Scientist: The billboard is made up of light bulbs that flash off and

---

[8]Davidson, D.: *Essays on Actions and Events* (Oxford, Clarendon Press, 1980). See the essay, "Mental Events" (p. 207).

on. Suppose you studied one light bulb in one corner over time. You could tell us how often the bulb was on and how long it was off. But you could not tell us what the bulb participated in, for example, a picture of a camel's foot. Your view is too close up to grasp the overall picture at a higher level. Studying neurons will tell us a lot about neurons, but a study of larger aggregates is needed to tell us what is going on at the higher level of mental activity. A single neuron can be participating at one moment in speaking French and at another moment in selecting a chess move. Just as with the Camel ad sign, we must widen neurophysiological perspectives.

Inquirer: You admit mental processes are properties of brains, or at least central nervous systems, and brains are composed of assemblies of cells, in turn made up of atoms. So why then cannot mental processes be eventually reduced to physics or chemistry?

Mind
Scientist: You are still confusing compositional constitutive properties with other sorts of properties. A book is certainly composed of atoms. The ink marks on its pages have a chemistry. But the marks stand for words in a language; they are signs, representations, symbolic properties of the book that result from human mental processes.[9] The meaning of the message does not lie in the chemistry of the ink. One can study and work out concepts, kinds, laws, and theories of symbolic properties (e.g. the grammar of language) without having to bring in knowledge of chemical or physical properties. It is not that physics and chemistry are not relevant to the existence of the book, but that *knowledge* of physical and chemical kinds and laws is not directly relevant to

---

[9]Peirce divided signs into icon, index, and symbol. An iconic sign looked like what it stands for, as does a stick figure a man or a curve on a road sign. An index is physically connected to an X and calls attention to X but does not describe X. A knock on the door is an example of an index. A symbol describes, stands for, and represents X without looking like it. As a proxy, it stands for X. The symbol "apple" does not look like an apple. Mental representations are symbolic proxies, codifications. Cf. Peirce, *Collected Papers* (2:247). For ages philosophers mistakenly believed that the mind actually mirrored nature rather than codifying it. A contemporary criticism of this glassy-essence misconception can be found in Rorty, R.: *Philosophy and the Mirror of Nature* (Princeton, Princeton University Press, 1979).

understanding the book's symbolic properties.[10]

Symbols are not deducible from a theory of atoms and hence are not reducible to an atom-and-the-void theory, if by reduction you mean deducible consequence. A deduction may still not provide an explanation of how a system works. Higher levels do not deny objects of lower levels; they enrich lower levels with novel and radical assumptions, properties, data, etc.[11] If a reductionist claims that he can predict symbolic properties, such as the meaning of a sentence, from neurophysiological or neurochemical principles, then instead of wasting a lot of our time arguing, let him produce the reduction so it can be evaluated. Otherwise reductionist claims are diaphanous. They represent vaporific froth, the verbal flourishes of hand-waving, a polite term in artificial intelligence for bullshitting.

Inquirer: You said you were not going to spend much time on the problem of reduction.

Mind
Scientist: My argument runneth over. I have found that people like yourself with a purely matterist training in medicine have a hard time getting this problem of levels straight. They somehow think everything must be reducible to the concepts, kinds, laws and vocabulary of physics and that science is whatever physicists countenance at the moment.

Inquirer: Is there a crucial difference between the laws of physics and the laws of psychology?

Mind
Scientist: There exists a great variety of scientific laws and statements about them.[12] Laws can be causal, func-

---

[10]All signs are in part physical in that they are embodied in the physical form we call a signal. The sound waves of speech are transduced eventually into electrochemical signals of the central nervous system. These signals modulate the ongoing activity of neurons just as hormones or other chemical substances do. Some people continue to wonder how mental disorders can arise from both symbolic and chemical inputs. The symbolic is just as physical in causing effects as is the chemical. In *addition* to their physical properties, symbols possess a non-physical property of representing the content of messages. Mental activity depends on a symbol-matter system.

[11]See Bunge, M.: Emergence and the mind (*Neuroscience*, 2:501, 1977).

[12]See Kaplan, A.: *Conduct of Inquiry* (p. 104).

tional, theoretic, taxonomic. Law statments range from strict generalizations to tendency statements, taking forms such as:

All A's are B's.

Everything that is an A is also a B.

Whenever A is present, then B tends to be present.

These are dyadic relations between two kinds of objects or properties or states (e.g. "all fish are vertebrates," or "everything that is a whale is a mammal," or "whenever paresis is found, then brain spirochetes tend to be found"). In the cognitive sciences, we are studying people's internal representation or conceptual model of signs. The relation is triadic. We do not say "A signifies B," but "A signifies B to C" where C is an interpreter. The triad is irreducible, just as you cannot reduce "A gives B to C" to "A parts with B" and "C acquires B," because of the intentional act of giving of B is different from the accidental acquisition of B.[13]

Inquirer: But how are you going to formulate objective general laws in psychology about uniquely subjective interpreters, the C in your triad?

Mind
Scientist: Laws are generalizations whose central terms refer to kinds. Our kinds in the mind sciences are *kinds* of signs, *kinds* of representations, and *kinds* of interpreters. A preliminary taxonomy is involved just as in physics or chemistry. By "objectivity" I will mean a fixed intersubjectivity in which qualified members of an expert community agree on some aspect of a system during a time interval, regardless of an individual's personal preferences. I think we can strive for agreements about the kinds C who interpret kinds of signs, A, as signifying kinds of entities, B. Once this is done, you can attempt to bring members sharing characteristics under common principles, rules, or laws. It has been done, for example, in the case of the kind C in which the inter-

---

[13]He states the relation is triadic. Ordinary language statements such as these are polyadic because each word can have multiple meanings in multiple contexts.

preters are characterized as paranoid.[14]

The more controversial issues between natural and mental sciences concern problems of intention and interpretation. Eventually we want to explain and understand human behavior. The problem of intention we share with psychology and biology.[15] To explain some aspects of an animal's behavior, psychologists and biologists refer to intentions, to what an animal is *trying* to do to achieve a goal. Animals seem to us to be purposive systems engaging in goal-directed activities. We impute intentionalistic ascriptions to them of the sort, "A performs action X in order to achieve goal Y." In our intentionalistic idioms, animals pursue some objects and situations they construe as satisfying or valuable and avoid others that are not. These teleological explanations of purposive systems were long in disrepute, especially for classical mechanists who were made uneasy by the concepts of goal, purpose, and intention. Aristotle believed that inanimate objects have the intention of moving toward the earth. When Galileo showed the inadequacy of this type of explanation for the freefall of objects, it was thought all teleological or purposive explanations had been discredited.[16] Not all systems are purely mechanical systems. In dealing with living organisms, the concepts of goal, purpose, and valued and disvalued outcomes are still indispensible.

---

[14]This model, exemplifying the kind "paranoia," will be discussed and debated quite soon.

[15]For a comprehensive treatment of the problem in psychology, see Boden, M.: *Purposive Explanation in Psychology* (Cambridge, Harvard University Press, 1972). In biology, see Wright, L.: *Teleological Explanations* (Berkeley, University of California Press, 1976).

[16]What Galileo showed was that physical objects falling towards the earth are not usefully viewed as instances of a purposive system. A theoretical system stipulatively specifies the design of a *kind* of schematic, simplified, idealized hypothetical system intended to have applications to *kinds* of empirical systems under some description or characterization. The relation between the two is an informal set-theoretic predicate "is an instance of." A kind of empirical system is an instance of (to some degree of approximation) the theoretical system that provides standards against which empirical observations can be compared and adjustments made. When it is decided from back-and-forth experience with the relations between the two systems that aspects of the empirical systems do not satisfy the specifications of the theoretical system, it is only the set-theoretic predicate that is falsified (i.e. the theoretical system does not apply to this particular empirical system), although it may have other applications of any degree of generality. This is why it makes little sense to claim that a deliberately simplified sketchy, idealized, postulated

→

Inquirer: Perhaps an animal does not have a goal, whatever "have" means. To us, from the outside, it looks as if he had a goal because the directive correlations between his actions and their objects are far greater than chance coincidence. If a chicken pecks at a grain of corn directly in front of him, and we move the grain of corn to the right, he turns himself to the right to peck again directly in front of himself. He does not go on pecking in his original position. It is "as if" he has a goal of pecking the corn which remains invariant under transformations of the spatial location of the particular grain of corn.[17] The "as if" serves as a convenient explanatory and successfully predictive device constructed by us humans. It may be in part a metaphor not to be taken entirely literally. We say an animal "has the goals of survival and reproduction." But it is implausible to me that there exist instructions in an animal's program that say "SURVIVE" and "REPRODUCE YOURSELF."

Mind
Scientist: Such high-level instructions in a program may not be necessary. It is not implausible that some animals contain internally pre-wired instructions such as "SEEK X" and "AVOID Y" that, when executed by a supervisory program, result in their survival. The factors X and Y are not literally goal situations but *concepts* or representations of goal situations which serve a control function

---

theoretical system is true or false. It has epistemic utility in solving problems or it does not.

Once, we believed the solar system was an instance of a Newtonian particle system. Now we believe it is an instance of an Einsteinian particle system that holds to a higher order of approximation. But an atomic system is not considered to be an instance of an Einsteinian particle system because, in addition to gravitational forces, electromagnetic forces are involved. Thus, theories are not conclusively proved true or false; they are simply replaced, dislodged or abandoned as outmoded for certain purposes if they do not epistemically apply in solving problems. Classical Newtonian mechanics is still good enough to build bridges but not to build neutron bombs. It has not been discredited. Its scope has become limited but not its application for certain purposes. To navigate ships and planes, we still apply Ptolemy's system that assumes the sun moves around the earth. If you have the mathematics for it, consult Sneed, J. D.: *The Logical Structure of Mathematical Physics* (Holland, Dordrecht, 1971), or Stegmüller, W.: *The Structure and Dynamics of Theories* (New York, Springer Verlag, 1976). For a simpler account, see Giere, R.: *Understanding Scientific Reasoning* (New York, Holt, Rinehart, and Winston, 1979).

[17]The corn-pecking chicken example is from Sommerhoff, G.: *Logic of the Living Brain* (New York, John Wiley, 1974).

in the choice of actions leading to favorable or un-
favorable outcomes. When do we move from metaphor
to literalness? At some point in the stages of science, we
decide our hypotheses are no longer metaphors but have
literal interpretations in real systems. Why not now take
the plunge and assume people carry internal structures
conceptually representing preferred human goals and
that such structures are involved in producing informed
courses of action? Note that I contrast informed courses
of action with reflexes and such actions as glomerular
filtration by the kidneys.

Inquirer: Couldn't these intentional structures be "reduced" to
some sort of mechanism?

Mind
Scientist: This is what a current argument in the behavioral sciences is all about when it comes to explaining
human action. Classical mechanists want to explain informed action in terms of, say, neurophysiological
mechanisms, whereas others claim intention is irreducible in this way.[18] In my not-so-humble view, the solution lies in a broadened definition of mechanism. One
can speak of mechanisms in any domain from physical
to sociological. There is a mechanism for running a
clock, and there is a mechanism for electing a president.
The mechanisms involved in the mental activity of
humans are computational, not the free-fall or push-
pull mechanisms of a classical Newtonian particle
system. Computational mechanisms are mechanisms,
but they are not purely mechanical, if you see the
difference.

Informed human action is governed by rules, patterns, and strategies systematized in an internal model.
To understand a person's actions is to understand how
his model works; for instance, understanding the message

---

[18]Cf. Fodor, J. A.: *The Language of Thought* (New York, Crowell, 1975) for some further
difficulties in correlating specific mental activities with specific neurophysiological
mechanisms. Also, see Fodor, J. A.: *Representations: Philosophical Essays on the Foundations of
Cognitive Science* (Cambridge, MIT Press, 1981). Even if the "ultimate" explanations were cast
in neurophysiological terms one would still need mental predicates to describe and
characterize what it is that is being explained. See Harre, R.: *The Principles of Scientific Thinking*
(Chicago, University of Chicago Press, 1970, p. 203).

content of his set of inference rules for producing beliefs. The model must be described not as a set of numbers (which is not rich enough) but in language suitable for specifying the signification of messages. This is the perspective of contemporary artificial intelligence.[19] Its virtue is (1) that it satisfies the scientific requirement of publicly criticizable symbol-processing mechanisms that can be realized in a set of physical mechanisms and (2) that it includes intentionalistic concepts characteristic of teleological explanation.

Inquirer: How do you determine if this sort of physical-purposive viewpoint is applicable to, or fruitful for, problems of mental activity?

Mind
Scientist: The strategy of contemporary artificial intelligence (AI) is constructive and compositional. It starts with whole behaviors, analyzes them into components, and then tries to put the components together in the form of a computational model. The strategy is guided by an idealized theoretical system and involves building things, both out of substances and out of symbols. It involves what AI jargon calls a "top-down" strategy, in contrast to the "bottom-up" strategy of traditional psychology that has tried to start with simple units and then build them up into systems which account for complex phenomena.[20] The top-down strategy of AI is transcendental in the original Kantian sense. It starts with the question, "What will a system have to have in order to accomplish X or to produce the behavior pattern Y? Starting with higher-level and more abstract units, AI workers try to put things together into a model, an algorithm, a computer program, and then see how the algorithm works when it is run as a model, an empirical system embodying a theoretical system. Initially, one evaluates the result with simple face

[19]See Boden, M.: *Artificial Intelligence and Natural Man* (New York, Basic Books, 1977). For the educated reader, this book offers the best introduction to some of the innards of artifical intelligence.
[20]A philosopher sympathetic to the efforts of AI describes this strategy in further detail in Dennett, D. C.: *Brainstorms: Philosophical Essays on Mind and Psychology* (Vermont, Bradford Books, 1978).

validity. Does the model do what it is supposed to do? Does it reproduce, to some acceptable degree of empirical approximation, the behavior under study? Does the interaction of the model's components perform the functions its theory explains? Does it achieve the desired empirical effects?

We tend to believe we understand effects if we can produce them ourselves. When chemists synthesize insulin that shows some of the effects of natural insulin, the demonstration indicates that the chemist has an understanding of the structure of insulin. The determination of a successful production is ultimately made through perceptual judgments, the resource used in all sciences that obtain agreements about recognized patterns.[21] In electrodynamics, for example, does the pointer on a galvanometer point approximately, with some degree of tolerance, to where it should point as predicted by the theory? If so, we believe in the possibility that the theory applies. But if the observed pointer reading is too far away from the theoretically predicted pointer reading — and here expert judgments are needed to evaluatively decide what cannot be tolerated — something is wrong, either in the theory or in the procedure used for experimental observation. Similarly in AI research, we observe the input/output patterns of a model and decide whether the patterns, using evaluative decision rules, make the sense they should in terms of the taxonomic and explanatory theory involved. The observed patterns can be linguistic since a sentence is just as factual an object for pattern recognition as is a pointer reading. The reading of a number on a galvanometer requires expert interpretation, as does the reading of an utterance in a psychiatric interview.

Take PARRY, a computer model of a hypothetical paranoid patient, as an example.[22] Clinicians familiar

---

[21]See Polanyi, M.: *Personal Knowledge* (p. 98).

[22]For the most complete and up-to-date description of this paranoid model, accompanied by the commentary of peer reviewers and an unhesitant rebuttal, see Colby, K.M.: Modeling a paranoid mind (*Behavioral and Brain Sciences*, 4:515, 1981). See also Faught, W.S., Colby, K.M., and Parkison, R.C.: Inferences, affects, and intentions in a model of paranoia (*Cognitive Psychology*, 9:153, 1977).

with paranoid disorders — and this is a class of phenomena, a kind that is highly reliable in the sense of interjudge agreements — interviewed the model in natural language and judged it to be paranoid.[23] They recognize that (1) these are the sort of things paranoid patients say, (2) in this interview context, (3) in response to the sort of things psychiatrists say. The validity of the simulation bottoms out at the level of pattern recognition by relevant experts. The model instantiates paranoid phenomena and is judged by its effects. Its input/output patterns are not discordant with the patterns expert judges recognize as paranoid. A reason for espousing of this type of a model lies in its power to generate specific qualitative effects. Sentences manifesting a diversity of characteristic patterns are derivable from a stringent set of underlying patterns that conform to a few basic principles.

We build an empirical system, a new object in the form of a computational model hypothesized in accordance with a theoretical system to simulate other empirical systems (i.e. individuals of a natural kind). We then test it for its effects. The model itself does not make quantitative predictions. Sciences can make all sorts of predictions, but this success does not make the predictions intelligible. We want informative ordering principles that explain the known phenomena even if they cannot make new predictions. If a model generates behavior which has the effects on expert judges similar to those produced by patients, then we say it is a successful simulation model. Clinicians also have interviewed PARRY and an actual patient and were asked to judge which is which.[24] Since they could

---

[23]The reliability of the kind "paranoid" has been repeatedly shown to be high. See Spitzer, R. L., Forman, Y. B. W., and Nee, J.: op. cit., as well as Kendler, K. S.: The nosologic validity of paranoia (simple delusional disorder) (*Archives of General Psychiatry, 37*:699, 1980). The properties of the kind "paranoia" described by Kendler are the manifest properties exhibited by the model PARRY.
[24]For the details of this experiment, see Heiser, J., Colby, K.M., Faught, W.S., and Parkison, R.C.: Can psychiatrists distinguish a computer simulation of paranoia from the real thing? The limitations of Turing-like tests as measures of the adequacy of simulation (*Journal of Psychiatric Research, 15*:149, 1980). Turing's test is an old war-horse in AI. The →

not clearly distinguish model from patient, we conclude, on the basis of empirical indiscernibility that the model, although a crude beginning, represents a satisfactory first-order coarse approximation and simulation of paranoid behavior.

Inquirer: That doesn't mean the internal workings of the model are necessarily the same as, or similar to, the internal workings of a paranoid patient.

Mind
Scientist: The relations between theories and models are a bit too long-winded for the purposes of our discussion here. Let me offer only a skeletal synopsis to answer your question. When the input/output behaviors of a simulation model successfully imitate those of a class or kind of empirical systems, we can say they are manifestly similar or equivalent in their effects at the level of empirical observation just as gravitational and inertial mass are equivalent in their effects on material objects. Next comes the problem of a theoretical structural equivalence at the level of unobservable mechanisms generating the characteristic input/output behavior. By "structure" here I am not referring to a material structure but to an organization or system of internal functions or processes. How is the successful manifest simulation or imitation produced? In the paranoid model, it is produced by an underlying complex algorithm consisting of a system of specific interdependent computational procedures that are postulated to be functionally analogous to the computational procedures

---

general idea involves an ability of human judges to distinguish a man from a machine programmed to behave like a man in response to interview questions. Thousands of articles have been written on the subject since 1950. Much of the debate is summarized in Colby, 1981, Modeling a paranoid mind (1981, p. 530). See also Hofstadter, D. R.: The Turing test: a coffeehouse conversation. In Hofstadter, D. R., and Dennett, D. C. (Eds.): *The Mind's I: Fantasies and Reflections of Self and Soul* (New York: Basic Books, 1981). This volume represents a collection of easy-to-read articles on many of the issues surrounding artificial intelligence and computational models of mental processes.

   Leibniz proposed a principle of indiscernibility of identicals or its converse, the identity of indiscernibles. It depends on what level the discerning is taking place. Two pencils may not be discernible to the naked eye, but become so in inspecting them with a magnifying glass. Leibniz meant that if all the properties of X and Y are identical, then X and Y are identical. Models are not identical with their subject matter in this sense.

used by the paranoid class of empirical systems under study. By functional analogy, I mean the computational processes play abstract roles in the model similar to their counterparts in the patient. The analogy is formal, not substantive; the sameness or similarity consists of the same abstract jobs being done. The regularities in the model correspond to, or are mirrored in, their counterpart regularities in the patient; they perform the same computational work.

In making the identifications between processes in the model and their counterparts in the patient, we do not claim they are truly "identical," but we treat them as if they were in this context and for our purposes. A theoretical system consists of a set of specifications for an idealized kind of empirical system, and linkages are made by epistemic correlations or coordinating definitions between propositions describing the two systems.[25] The actual empirical systems that the theoretical system can be applied to are the models of the theory, empirical systems that approximately satisfy the theory's specifications. Thus, PARRY and paranoid patients, in the sense they are physical realizations, are models of the theoretical system specified for actual paranoid systems.

This theory contains a proto-law, a generalization as stated in this conditional probabilistic formula:

If either C_1 or C_2 or C_3. . . Cn, then PA is likely in virtue of P_1 and P_2 and P_3 and . . . Pn.

In this law-like statement, the Cs represent an open disjunction of clinically well-known situations that precipitate paranoid states such as birth of a deformed child, false arrest, increasing deafness, Wernicke's aphasia. The letters PA stand for the properties characteristic of the "natural" kind *paranoia*. The Ps represent an open conjunction of information processes specified by the theory as the underlying causal generating mechanisms or strategies responsible for

---

[25]The specifications describe the initial state of they system. They do not describe how the system got to be that way. Thus, they are postulates to be taken as starting points to see where we can get from this initial stance.

manifest paranoid phenomena. The explanatory theory posits a stringent set of underlying patterns able to unify a great diversity of manifest patterns whose descriptions are derivable from the common generative patterns shared by members of the kind *paranoid*. The disjunctions and conjunctions are open, in that future discoveries may add to them as well as to the descriptions of the paranoid mode. Also, I should emphasize that the formula proposes only sufficient and not necessary conditions and carries the probabilistic rider "likely."

Inquirer: Why do you call the theory "explanatory"?

Mind
Scientist: Because of its ability to unify very heterogeneous facts that are difficult to connect and understand otherwise. It makes a range of seemingly disparate phenomena intelligible by grouping and uniting them under an underlying core of causal patterns of information processing. Common sense is hard put to see any connection at all between false arrest and the birth of a defective child in the production of paranoid reactions. A good explanation is surprise-reducing, in that by unification, coherent sense is made out of otherwise inexplicable connections. To say someone is paranoid is to say that he is as a member of a natural kind. An explanatory theory describes why he does what he does under certain circumstances. A theory explains when it entails a description of the already known phenomena that pose the problem.

The important point here is that PARRY has been created as an empirical system with the help of the theory, whereas paranoid patients are "naturally occurring" examples. PARRY is an empirical system of existential novelty that no one ever thought of artificially producing before. The network of internal components and their structured relations in the model represent a demonstratively actual and credibly possible way paranoid behavior can be generated, in contrast to a merely conceivably possible way. The model is consistent, compatible and nondiscordant with clinical observations. It "predicts" the known phenomena in that they are derivable from the generative structure of the model. Science pursues the possibles and rejects the impossibles more than it makes final conclusions about the "truth."[26] The observed linguistic patterns PARRY are derivable consequences from the internal patterns of model which is the least one expects of a good model.

Remember, the model *can fail*; it is refutable. It could be deemed *not* an instance of paranoid interview behavior. If the model were *not* diagnosed paranoid and if it *were* distinguished from an actual patient, we would say something is inadequate about the model or about the experimental setup. Science is not so much trial and error, but an informed try, fail, and try again. We can tell when a model is not working the way it should (i.e. not making sense) by using our pattern-recognition judgments. But when the model does work "correctly," all we can say, at this stage, is that this is a credible system of mechanisms for an explanation of the underlying processes involved in producing the phenomena.[27] It is not that paranoia *must* work this way; it *may* work this way as a first approximation. The model PARRY instantiates (is an individual instance of) the kind of empirical phenomena we term *paranoid*. To strengthen our belief in the applicability of the theory underlying the algorithm, we need further tests of the model as well as empirical tests of the theory embodied in the model.

Inquirer: What sort of empirical tests?

Mind
Scientist: The theory realized as a model in PARRY posits struc-

---

[26]Another philosophical treatment of AI along these lines can be found in Sloman, A.: *The Computer Revolution in Philosophy: Philosophy, Science, and Models of Mind* (New York, Humanities Press, 1978).
[27]A functional class is one whose members produce objects/actions of a specific type. Members of the class are not identical but equivalent with respect to object/action types produced. Manifest functional equivalence between model and patient means resemblance in performance in that the macrostructure of input/output behavior of the two systems is similar. Turing-like tests are ways of estimating the similarities and dissimilarties; they justify the simulation and they test the applicability of the theoretical system embodied in the model. Structural equivalence means that the internal microstructures and processes posited in the theoretical system and realized in the model correspond to, or parallel, their counterparts in a paranoid patient. Tests for this strong form of structural equivalence are hard to come by. Cf. Colby, Modeling a paranoid mind (1981, p. 531).

tures and processes that attempt to reduce the distress induced by the affect of shame-humiliation triggered by the activations of self-defectiveness beliefs. If one had a measure of the affect of shame, such as increased blood flow in the ear lobes and its accompanying rise of temperature, that we know occurs during moments of experienced shame, one could compare measured values of paranoid patients and non-patients under experimental shame-inducing conditions. If we had a drug that raised the threshold of shame, such as we have for anxiety, such a drug would help paranoid conditions. This treatment-response prediction is a derivable consequence of the shame-theory of paranoid systems. Or, as another test, we could compare the frequency of paranoid disorders in cultures utilizing shaming techniques for socialization versus the frequency of paranoid disorders in cultures which make little use of these techniques. I cite these examples merely to illustrate that AI theories can be tested in ways additional to model-building and model-testing, and thus AI can be science-extending because the implication of its theories fan out in many directions to gain empirical anchorage.

Inquirer: Let's charitably assume a successful simulation model as a first approximation provides a faint plus in favor of the theory it realizes. What about other existing theories of paranoid phenomena? Using the Schreber case, Freud thought homosexual conflict was the basis of paranoia. In today's preferred jargon, we would classify Schreber's concerns as transsexual rather than homosexual.[28] But there are an infinity of theories

---

[28]See Stoller, R. J.: *Sex and Gender: The Transsexual Experiment* (London, Hogarth, 1975). For a discussion of alternative theories of paranoia, see Colby, K. M.: An appraisal of four psychological theories of paranoia (*Journal of Abnormal Psychology*, 86:54, 1977). The upshot of this discussion is that current rival theory candidates can be viewed as special cases of the theory realized in the paranoid model PARRY. As Kuhn has emphasized, there exists no universal decision rule that scientists use for theory choice. See Kuhn, op. cit. This does not imply the preference by scientists of one theory over another is irrational. The decisions involve relations between empirical system data and their approximation to the standards concluded from the principles of the hypothesized theoretical system. What principles are

→

which might entail or be consistent with the data.

Mind
Scientist: People trained in mathematics like to talk this way
because they have been taught that an infinite number
of curves can be drawn between data points on a graph.
The concept of infinity seems to have an infinite number
of meanings. But ours is a small infinity in the factual
sciences where it is sometimes difficult to think up even
one plausible theory. How many alternative theories of
evolution are there? It is very hard to think up alternatives
to Euclidean geometry which began as a metaphor.[29]
There are only eight to ten theories of gravitation taken
seriously and only five or six are considered viable in that
models can be constructed from them.

If someone has a different theory of the processes
underlying paranoid phenomena, let him build a model
of it and show it to us. The model should be an
algorithm specified in a programming language if we
are to have initial consensibility and affirmability. Now
we compare descriptions of the rival models. Are the
models really different? There are many constraints
which must be respected if the input/output patterns
observed are to be judged typical of paranoia. Are these
constraints so strong that the new model is not really
different in principle but just another way (e.g. nota-
tional) of saying the same thing? If the new model cannot pass the simplest test (i.e. being diagnosed
paranoid), we should drop it as a viable alternative. To
paraphrase Sherlock Holmes, if we eliminate the impossibles, what we wind up with, however improbable,
is a $truth_2$. Or I would temper the jargon to say, we
wind up with a small candidate set of interpretations for
$truth_2$.

Remember, $truth_2$ is not a property of the theory but

---

involved in theory choice itself remain unknown. Among eligible rival theories, the preferred
theory is often the one that has a wider umbrella of consequences and that best unifies the
phenomena characteristic of the natural kinds involved.
[29]See Klein, op. cit. Most of us, even today, take Euclidean, three-dimensional empty space,
not as a metaphor, but as literally true. In physics, there are now about ten different
geometries being used.

of the set-theory predicate stating that the empirical system is an instance of the theoretical system. We can rely on one or the other of the candidate theories in guiding our actions, depending on our purposes and the sorts of technological or pragmatic problems we are trying to solve. In time, one candidate theory might win out as the most applicable. Or maybe the whole candidate set will be abandoned as inadequate and a new one generated. But I'll bet any new one in the next few years will involve computational functions because they are the sort of mechanisms that can produce the phenomena and that do justice to the theoretical complexity of mental activity.

Inquirer: All we have to do is to clarify this new concept of computational function as a non-push-pull mechanism.

Mind
Scientist: That is the task of contemporary and future students of mental processes. We try to understand phenomena, not only by finding out what kinds of things exist, but also by trying to make new things exist, like computational models. Artificial intelligence as theoretical psychology starts with the representation problem. We presuppose humans retain internal representations of their past experience. The lowest-level internal representation of signs is abstract and unique. For example, when you look at a book, multiple representations can occur on the retina as you turn the book around, or look at it upside down, or under different degrees of light. However, your internal representation consists of factored-out enduring constants, or invariances, in contrast to the multiple subjective ephemeral representations on the retina. This does not mean that the content of your unique representation of the objective features of an object exactly matches the content of mine in all details. But there is a consonance or match or commonality or similarity between our representational contents which allows us to talk about and successfully manipulate both symbols and objects similarly. These abstract and factored-out representations can be transformed into still other, higher-level representations.

The representations are representations to somebody and are used by the agent purposively. Representations do not just sit there; they are functional, they *do* things. They play a causally efficacious role in determining human action just as much as does, say, a low blood-sugar or high blood-alcohol. A system that can be aware of products of its own representational activity can be said to possess a type of consciousness.

Inquirer: Hold it! That would imply that a computer programmed to have representation of itself within itself could be conscious. But surely we wouldn't want to call it conscious. You must be using the term in a special way.

Mind
Scientist: That I am. By this type of consciousness, I do not mean being awake. To describe a comatose patient, physicians say he is "unconscious," meaning he is not awake. I have a specific sense for the term. Let's start with a concept of awareness somewhat different from that ordinarily used. We confidently attribute the property of awareness to animals because they make discriminations necessary for an appropriate directively correlated response to objects in their environment. Recall the chicken and his grain of corn of a few moments ago. We do not just attribute, we are *convinced* we humans possess such awareness. By "self-awareness," I will mean to be aware of, to notice, to detect discriminations about oneself as distinct from other entities. Besides noticing objects, and ourselves, we notice what we "think" *about* them (i.e. we are "L-conscious"). I am restricting the term *L-conscious* to a particular subset of self-awareness in which we have access to mental products in linguistic speech form.[30] The "speech" we notice and attend to is our own inner speech.

Inquirer: How does your position differ from Sperry's? Sperry

---

[30]Some, but not all, of these conceptual distinctions are drawn in Dennett, D. C.: *Content and Consciousness* (New York, Humanities Press, 1969, p. 114), and in Dennett: *Brainstorms* (1978, p. 149). Dennett does not consider L-consciousness as a special kind of self-awareness, but he might. He defines being "aware₁" as awareness of mental input to a "speech center," thus opening the door to the idea of a suitably programmed machine being L-conscious, if it had a speech center. Here, L-consciousness refers to *output* from an inner speech center. We will use the general term *linguistic* to open the door further to computers that can only "read" products of their mental activity instead of "hearing" them as inner speech. The linguistic expressions in L-consciousness are vehicles for underlying representations. See Rosenberg, J.: *Linguistic Representation* (Dordrecht-Holland, Reidel, 1972).

seems to believe that consciousness, as an emergent property, has a causal influence on brain processes.[31]

Mind
Scientist: I have always been sympathetic towards Sperry's stance on this issue because, using my own computational analogy and vocabulary, I think I knew what he was getting at, even though he has been subjected to all sorts of name-calling that scientists use, such as mystical and animistic. If we can straighten out a few terminological snarls and use some different analogies, I think his position would be more acceptable to contemporary cognitive scientists. It is his statement that conscious mental processes influence brain processes that sticks in the craw. It sounds dualist, but it is really monist with levels of description being mixed, in which a taxonomic relation, such as mental processes to brain processes, is being confused with a causal relation. To avoid mixing taxonomic and causal levels of descriptions, Sperry should say that conscious mental contents causally influence subsequent mental processes. Mental processes are supervenient upon and *depend* on brain processes, but mental processes influence mental processes and brain processes influence other brain processes. If we don't keep these levels straight, we get into all kinds of clouded and needless arguments.

Instead of Sperry's analogy of the size and shape of a rolling wheel determining the fate of its constituent atoms and molecules, a better, although purely mechanical, analogy would be that of an induction motor that generates a magnetic field which, in turn, effects the behavior of the induction motor. Both entities are "material" or "physical," but they are in different phases of "matter" having different properties.

Inquirer: But something is missing in the analogy. If conscious mental content is not physical or material, how can it act back on something material like brain processes?

---

[31]See Sperry, R. W.: An objective approach to subjective experience: further explanation of a hypothesis (*Psychological Review, 77*:585, 1970). Cf. also his In search of psyche. In Worden, F., Swazey, J. P., and Adelmans, I. (Eds.): *The Neurosciences: Paths of Discovery* (Cambridge, MIT Press, 1975, p. 425), and also Mind-brain interactions: mentalism, yes; dualism no (*Neuroscience, 5*:195, 1980). His latest treatment is *Science and Moral Priority: Merging Mind Brain, and Human Values* (New York, Columbia University Press, 1983).

| Mind Scientist | That is why I said the induction-motor analogy is purely mechanical. It lacks the additional power of symbols in a symbol-matter system. The contents of L-consciousness are symbolic signs. Signs are just as physical as anything else, but, in addition, they have symbolic properties of being messages in a code. A better symbol-processing analogy for Sperry would be a computer system that, in reading its own output in English, reacts to this output and modifies its subsequent behavior. The modification first requires the translation from the higher-level language of English to the machine-language level in which there is finally a one-to-one correspondence between the symbols of a bit pattern and a pattern of electromagnetic fields. |

Reading the English output would be analogous to our experiencing conscius mental content in linguistic forms. In Sperry's terms, the "higher order" organization or phase of ordinary linguistic description has a directive control function on transconscious mental processes, but only when it is fed back into the system's cycles and gets translated into a different phase or code of "lower order" machine languages where direct causal relations occur between bit patterns and electromagnetic fields. I would propose that mental processes as signs, and brain processes as electrochemical reactions, are *both* instances of different *phases* of the basic stuff of the universe, which ultimately is simply information. Of course, this is a purely metaphysical belief.

| Inquirer: | If I were a strict materialist, I would say that certain brain processes generate something like an electromagnetic field that we experience as conscious qualities. My analogy would be that in conscious perception we experience the color red, but we know that what we call "redness" stems from the impingement of electromagnetic waves of a certain wavelength on our retina. |

| Mind Scientist: | Your analogy is tenable as long as you remember that your conscious experience of "redness" is the composite product of electromagnetic waves and your own inner |

workings as a particular organism and person that result in the final product of what you label a color. Also, I must warn you about being a materialist. For some people, material or matter means that which has mass. But fields have no mass. If you widen the definitions of matter to include fields, then you leave room for a concept of matter having different phases with different properties in each phase so that the laws of one phase do not necessarily apply across a phase boundary to another phase. The phases may have law-like symmetry connections, however. In a computer system, the higher order phase of symbols of the program, given suitable translation into machine language code, govern the lower order phase of the input-output behavior of the machine that is harnassed in the service of the program. I think this is what Sperry has been trying to get at.

Inquirer: How does your defintion of L-consciousness differ from the traditional concept of introspection?

Mind Scientist: They are roughly synonymous, with one additional distinction. I would say L-consciousness or introspection is awareness at time t of symbols resulting from mental processes that *have already* taken place at a previous time t-1. We are not L-conscious of mental processes themselves, only of their results. In one sense, the expressed contents of introspection are retrospected since the non-linguistic production of the contents has already occurred. The L-consciousness or introspection itself, however, occurs at time t. Retrospection about what I was L-conscious of yesterday obviously involves memory functions.

Inquirer: Suppose I am L-conscious in the sense of being aware of some results of my own mental activity. I have access to these results displayed to me in auditory linguistic form. What good does that do me? What is this access consciousness for? What does it do?

Mind Scientist: Two things. First, L-consciousness is a means for linguistic communication of mental products, say, ideas, with others as well as with oneself. To tell others what you think, you must be aware of at least part of what you think. Second, to induce oneself to change, one must have some communicative contact, some access to a description, of what it is that requires changing.[32] We conduct a dialogue with ourselves, with the topic under discussion being described to us in linguistic form. Notice, therefore, that what we detect and attend to in L-consciousness is under some description; it is a characterization.[33]

Inquirer: This is getting a bit thick.

Mind
Scientist: I regret it, but psychology is hard, despite the fact that undergraduates consider its courses "Mickey Mouse." I will repeat, awareness is a capacity to detect or notice signs. I take it for granted that to respond to signs appropriately, one must be aware of them as distinct from something else. Discriminated signs lead to the production of specific effects such as external actions. As systems, we can be aware of signs without being L-conscious of them. You are not L-conscious of most of the signs impinging on your sensors at this very moment.

L-consciousness represents a specific kind of access, of self-awareness, in which the signs noticed are particular symbolic products of our mental processes displayed and described in the linguistic auditory mode. We cannot detect *how* they are produced, only *that* they can be noticed by what has been traditionally called

---

[32]See Dennett, *Brainstorms* (1978, p. 285).

[33]The pronouns, *I, we, one, ourselves,* and *oneself* are being used here loosely in the idiom of a first-person language. "I" is a deictic label for a person. Although our criminal law looks at it this way, a person is not an agent that controls his mind and body; he *is* his mind and body. We use an "it" language to divide a person into parts and process. In an "it" language that involves parts and processes of the underlying representational system, two levels of the system must be involved. One level, the object system, carries out the first-order processing. A second level, the meta system, using second-order processing, monitors whether the first-level is succeeding. The meta system has second-order beliefs, desires, etc., regarding the object's system first-order beliefs, desires, etc. The object system is indicative; the meta system is normative about what should happen. Thus, the dialogue conducted within ourselves is between one system and another not between two homuncular persons within a person. The topic is too complicated to go into further for the purposes of this monograph. For a technical discussion of the functioning of meta and object systems, see Colby, Modeling a paranoid mind (1981, p. 526). The reason L-consciousness is being discussed at all there is because it bears directly on a proposed taxonomy of psychiatric patients to be outlined by the Grantsman in Dialogue IX.

"introspection." These linguistic contents of L-consciousness can function to change or revise a cognitively penetrable representation, which in turn may, or may not, result in a change in output action. One must change our own representations or programs, we must first be conscious of their products and have some access to them. To reprogram ourselves, we must self-formatively change instructions using a high level language.[34]

Inquirer: Then animals are aware and self-aware but do not have the special self-awareness of L-consciousness in your sense because they do not detect products of their own mental activity described in a ligustic form.

Mind
Scientist: Correct, unless some animals have a rudimentary language that can be used this way. By correct, I do not mean these are *the* correct definitions. I mean these are the definitions we should use for our purpose of disentangling and clarifying how some of these processes operate.

Inquirer: You still have not answered by question about computer consciousness.

Mind
Scientist: You are being most patient. If you view L-consciousness as an ability that a system has to notice some of of its own

---

[34]These complexities of self-induced change requiring acces can be viewed as a difference between interpreted and compiled versions of a program. In running an interpreted version of a program, the supervision program translates each instruction into machine language, executes the instruction, translates the next one and so on. A compiled program is first translated in its entirety into machine language and then the instructions are executed one by one. For routine tasks performed repeatedly, the compiled version is faster and more efficient, but it cannot be changed in the high-level programming language as the interpreted version can.

When you first learn the tennis instruction "watch the ball," you repeatedly say this phrase to yourself (L-consciousness). In time, the instruction is stored away and you can be L-conscious of other instruction such as "play his backhand." You (i.e. you as a system) are now "automatically" watching the ball (awareness) without your being L-conscious of it. When you start missing the ball, you must return to fundamentals and tell yourself again to watch the ball until it becomes automatic again. Since you do not have access to the compiled version, you must revise the interpreted version of the program, which is then recompiled and replaces the old compiled version. Thus, you are able to change or revise a mental process that leads to a change in intentional output action. All this is discussed in a more detailed way in Colby, K. M.: A reprogrammable function of conscious linguistic content(*Cognition and Brain Theory*, 4:369, 1981). For a discussion of cognitive penetrability, see Pylyshyn, Z.: Computation and cognition (*Behavioral and Brain Sciences*, 3:111, 1980).

mental, symbolic products, then computers can be programmed to be L-conscious *in this sense.*

Inquirer: Aha! Now I have you. You said animals and humans had awareness. But they are alive. A computer is not alive, so how can it be L-conscious or even aware?

Mind
Scientist: It's true I said animals and humans had awareness. But I did not say *only they* had this property. Any system that can make the appropriate distinction between signs in order to respond appropriately can be said to be aware. Even Descartes realized there is no necessary connection between being conscious and being alive.[35]

Notice that I am always referring to distinctive content as being effective and not to be the capacity to *feel* or to *experience* the content, which is obviously different in living and nonliving systems because they represent matter in very different phases and forms. Signs make us aware of *what they signify*, not of their physical media.

Inquirer: I fail to see the point. Aren't we aware of sound waves?

Mind
Scientist: We are, but it is not *their* structure we detect but the structure of the message being carried by them. Consider a phone call. When I talk to you on the phone, you are aware of, and respond to, the structure of my message, not to the mass-energy structure of the copper wire carrying the message. I could send you smoke signals, or flash a mirror, or write you communicating the same message. If the message stated that a large brush fire is approaching your property, you would react in the same way regardless of the message's physical medium. We are not aware of light waves but of rattlesnakes. What signs signify requires interpretation.

Inquirer: I still think it is a bit odd to speak of computer systems as having a type of consciousness. Also, I have a hard time separating the *experiencing* of L-consciousness from

---

[35]Sooner or later, in all extended discussions of mind, Descartes crops up. He has enlightened and confused us for centuries. One of his books, begun in 1628 but published after his death in 1650, had the engaging title *Rules For the Direction of the Mind.* It is not at all well-known that he broke the entailment between being conscious and being alive. Cf. Descartes, R.: *Treatise of Man*, trans. T. S. Hall (Cambridge, Cambridge University Press, 1972, p. 112).

its contents. I will have to ponder it further by myself. You said that what signs signify requires interpretation, and interpretation was your third problem regarding the natural and mental sciences. How does the problem of interpretation enter all of this?

Mind
Scientist: The hardest comes last. What makes psychology hard is not just that interpretations are involved. As the Metaphysician told us, there is an interpretative element in the simplest perception. What he did not tell you about are the double, triple, and even multiple interpretations involved in understanding and explaining human action. He avoided the swamps and miasmas of what some call "hermeneutics."

Inquirer: What in the world is hermeneutics?

Mind
Scientist: Hermeneutics is a theory of interpretation in philosophy. The word is derived from Hermes, the messenger of the gods who understood what gods said in their highfalutin language. Hermes translated from this language into terms ordinary mortals could understand. A translation of the god's messages was required because otherwise the god's meanings would be hidden from the common man. Early hermeneuticians were not only interpreters of the Bible but were considered infallible in their exegeses. Their readings represented what they would intend to mean if *they* wrote the biblical sentences. Although originally employed in literary and philosophical traditions to determine what a text "meant," nowadays the term often refers to interpreting any sort of signs generated by humans. One way of explaining human actions is to interpret its "meaning," a task whose practitioners the traditional natural scientist would certainly anathematize.

Inquirer: What is the natural scientist's objection to a concept of "meaning"?

Mind
Scientist: The term seems too imprecise and slippery for a science. It appears more often in literary rather than

scientific circles. But we have to come to terms with it. Rocks and clouds emit signs, but they do not send messages with meaning to one another as people do. In perceiving, we interpret signs. There are two sorts of signs, natural and deliberate. A certain cloud shape is a natural sign of rain to us humans. Because it is not a purposive system, a cloud itself is not an author of a sign intending to communicate a message to a second party. From our experience with the world, it is we who assign the message content of significance "rain" to our representation of the observed cloud.

A deliberate sign involves an author, an intention, and an intended second party towards whom the sign is directed. If I raise my hand in order to request that you stop talking, I have made a deliberate sign. Your interpretation of my sign as an intentional action carrying a message to stop talking would be correct in the sense that the significance you assigned to the message is the same as I, the author, assigned. However, you can simultaneously be reading other signs emanating from me as natural signs. For example, when I speak, I speak in English. It is not my purpose to communicate that I speak English, but you can interpret my doing so as a natural sign indicating linguistic competence in English. Given only this information, namely, that my hand went up, I don't think observers can decide which intentional interpretation is correct. An action is an intentional action *under some description*.[36] It is an instance of a *kind*. But which kind? My hand going up may signify a request to leave the room, a greeting to someone behind you, a yea-vote, etc. The action must be characterized as to its *kind* before we can offer an explanation of it in terms of a theoretical system. It is this characterization of kind I am calling "interpretation."

An interpretation assigns a significance to an action. To characterize an action one needs further information,

---

[36]See Anscombe, G. E. M.: *Intention*, 2nd ed (London, Blackwell. 1963), as well as Dennett, *Content and Consciousness* (1969, p. 156). Regarding signs, Heraclitus remarked, "The Lord whose oracle is at Delphi neither speaks nor conceals but gives signs."

more contextual facts, more data about the situation, including a person's own view of what he is doing. The interpretations of an agent's intentional messages readily become narrowed. In dealing with persons, it is an advantage to be a person oneself because we know what human intentional messages are like since we use them ourselves. In everyday life, we seem to arrive at hundreds and thousands of agreements about signs. We wouldn't survive a simple drive down a highway if we didn't. In principle, scientific agreements about patterns of human behavior are not impossible because, in so many contexts, we achieve consensus about message contents.

Inquirer: I don't see how other scientists could mount a strong argument against your position.

Mind
Scientist: Much depends on the scientists you hang around with. My own scientific colleagues in chemistry and biology have no trouble at all in talking about codes, information, signs, message content, etc. Information-processing theory provides a way of talking about molecules as being instructions as well as being just molecules. The letters DNA and RNA encode information in a way that simple H_2O does not. In taking DNA as analagous to a sentence, molecular biologists can show that some nucleotide triplets served as punctuation marks, signifying an end of message. I agree they seldom use the term *meaning*, but the analogy to *message content* is very close.

　　　Humans, at least sometimes, behave according to what a situation means for them, not necessarily in full accordance with the objective-to-others situation. Now here is where a double interpretation enters. First, a person, Observer I, who can observe products from his own mental activity interprets signs in a situation and responds to his construal with intentional actions. Then second, we as scientific observers, Observers II of Observer I, make an interpretation or characterization of his action that may or may not correspond to the agent's own interpretation, the meaning it has for *him*.

Inquirer: This is getting not only woolly, but hairy. How do you
              know what the agent's interpretation is to begin with?

Mind
Scientist: We agree that neither Observer I nor Observer II can
              directly observe mental activity. Observer I may be
              L-conscious of certain products, such as a linguistic
              description of the intention of his action. He can quote
              or paraphrase this description to Observer II using or-
              dinary language.[37]

Inquirer: But we know people are often mistaken about their own
              views of themselves. Self-deception, unconscious
              motivations, and misconceptions of situations can make
              subjective self-reports unreliable.

Mind
Scientist: But not always or totally unreliable. Mental states are
              not entirely or absolutely private. The signs an agent
              uses at any level are always incomplete since they are
              samples. The signs may be unrepresentative if they are
              biased samples. Actions as signs can be read by outside
              Observers II in two ways: (1) as signs of a mental
              state, or (2) as a manifestation of the state itself. Thus,
              complaining is not just a sign of discontent, it is also a
              manifestation of discontent. The inquiry doesn't end
              with a person's self-report. L-consciousness involves a
              type of observation of mental products, and, as we have
              seen, observation does not provide the entirely "hard"
              data it was once believed to. Even if L-consciousness
              reports are reliable, it does not entail they are incorrigi-
              ble or infallible. As Observers II, we must judge the
              agent's interpretation in the light of our own Observer
              II meaning system. We may decide the agent is
              "correct" or we may not. But what he tells us as self-
              knowledge about himself is one piece of contributory in-
              formation, one fact.

                    To lessen confusion, I will call Observer I's inter-

---

[37]In medieval terms, a direct quotation of a phrase or sentence is *oratio recta*. When the proposition underlying a sentence can be expressed in a number of ways, *oratio obliqua* becomes
employed. Errors can creep in anywhere along the line from the underlying *oratio obliqua* instructions to the *oratio recta* descriptions we "hear" in L-consciousness.

pretation of his action "interpretation" and Observer II's interpretation I will call "characterization." For Observers II, the characterization of an empirical system becomes the phenomena to be explained by the theoretical system. We need more information before we can arrive at the characterization to be explained.

Inquirer: This would seem to me to be a serious weakness of this approach. Suppose there is disagreement between agent, Observer I, and Observer II or between Observers II. How do you verify that any interpretation of an action is a correct fact?

Mind
Scientist: Undoubtedly there are difficulties. Before we get to correctness of fact, let us consider the role of rational testing procedures. Knowledge in science is subjected to batteries of tests. They can be non-empirical tests of internal consistency or coherence with other justified knowledge. And they can be empirical tests in which, for example, theory statements are compared with observation statements. Notice that if theory statements and observation statements are to be compared, their *meanings* must be coherent.

In our domain, the observations, the data, are signs with meaning emanating from human agents, the signs being samples of internal representations. A sign such as a word or phrase does not fully represent its concept. It is an abbreviation for a much larger network of structural relations. The signs we observe consist of intentional non-linguistic or linguistic actions and, I am suggesting, we add the agent's own interpretations of these actions. We, the Observers II, read these signs and messages in various ways depending on the purposes of our investigation. Our first purpose is to characterize and taxonomize actions and our second is to explain them. We can read actions as indicators of the agent's meaning and intentions, or we can read them as signs of other kinds (e.g. people with the ability to use correct plurals in English).

This is weakly analogous to reading Shakespeare,

where we can enjoy our own interpretations of what the author meant without worrying about what he himself intended to mean. But in the mind sciences, we usually want to discover what the agent intends to mean by his signs. It is subjective information, but we aim to explain the subjective objectively. When the readings of Observers II differ, we first must decide whether the characterizations are equisignificant and equivalent or represent genuinely conflicting accounts of the "facts." Suppose they are conflicting rivals. In the natural sciences, an appeal is made to other facts and to coherence. But even then, there are no brute facts independent of an interpretative element, and no single fact confirms or infirms. A concatenation of convergent evidence must be appealed to as the Biological Scientist asserted. The "facts of the matter" are part of the evidence.

Inquirer: What are the facts of the matter in the human case?

Mind
Scientist: Just as in the natural sciences, there is no ultimate fact, but there are multiple facts to be collected. The more we know about an individual, the more we can limit the possible characterizations of his actions and messages. A person can be operating under multiple controls or principles simultaneously. If we know his present and past history, his cultural upbringing, his environment, and facts about others like him including ourselves, we can conclude that when he waves his hand at us and says "Hi," he is offering a greeting. He is not exercising his mouth and hand muscles.

Inquirer: The example is simplistic and the characterization no better than those of ordinary folk psychology.[38]

Mind
Scientist: One can't be conclusive about it really. Any body of in-

---

[38]Folk psychology is nothing to be sneezed at for some purposes. It is invaluable for getting around in the world of other persons since it is quite successful, as measured by its predictive utility. For a further discussion of the virtues of folk psychology, see Churchland, P. M.: *Scientific Realism and the Plasticity of Mind* (Cambridge, Cambridge University Press, 1979), as well as Pylyshyn, Z.: Computation and cognition (*Behavioral and Brain Sciences, 3*:111, 1980).

formation does not determine a unique characterization. Consider the possibilities that have not even been thought of. A single action can have multiple correct readings because it satisfies multiple intentions running simultaneously in parallel. There will be different explanations for different constructs of signs. An absolute and final "God's truth" is too strong a criterion for science. A rough and ready justifiable truth$_2$ is good enough to get by on; it *satisfices*.[39] Many of my colleagues in psychology are preoccupied with a perfectionistic notion of truth they term *psychological reality*. For example, they expect the rules of a postulated grammar to be exactly the rules contained in human heads down to the last detail. But no theoretical system ever perfectly fits or entirely covers an empirical system it is applied to. The application needs only to be good enough to satisfy the absorbing concerns of the subject matter at a given time. Later, a better approximation will develop to fit both the old and new abiding concerns of a context.

The world itself eludes a definitive interpretation. Decisive, completely objective, neutral characterizations are impossible because observers have their own meaning systems. Science has an open context. Characterizations and explanations undergo revision and modification in the light of new knowledge. The best we can say, instead of TRUE, is that what we have is reasonably satisfactory or approximately correct provisionally for the time being and until further notice. All one might say is that a characterization or an explanatory theory is partially, approximately, and presumptively true because it is epistemically useful. Russell said the purpose of precise theory was to make approximations. Behind this quip lies the fact that to

[39]The term *satisfice* comes from decision theory. (Again, notice the affective aspect of scientific talk.) Operating under a number of constraints, decision-makers arrive at a decision that is satisfactory and suffices. It may not be optimal but it is tolerable and good enough under the given constraints. We will come across the term again in relation to mental health and mental disorder in Dialogue VIII.

confirm something as approximately true, one must assume other things to be actually true. But the circle is virtuous rather than vicious.

Inquirer: I think I follow only the gist of your rather arcane and winding argument. What does all this have to do with our problems in psychiatric taxonomy?

Mind
Scientist: Two things are relevant. First, the message is clear that you need additional novel properties to characterize patients with mental disorders. You find novel properties by having bright ideas about what they might be and through systematic research using new methods. I suggest you collect the patient's own interpretations, beliefs, or self-knowledge about himself and his condition, not just his symptoms, and look for patterns in this data. Second, perhaps you did not notice that I just said "others like him" in connection with constraining interpretations. This means constructing *kinds* of individuals who give similar *kinds* of interpretations of themselves. Such an investigation involves the whole domain of human mental activity. You are dealing with only a small subset of this domain — patients with mental disorders. Your task should be easier than ours because you are dealing with only a small subset of human kinds — those involving mental disorder.

Inquirer: Nothing is easy anymore. The easy problems are solved first. I will have to talk with someone in the domain of mental disorders who is also a psychologist and who is familar with diagnostic problems in psychiatry.

Mind
Scientist: Try the Clinical Pyschologist.

THE CLINICAL PSYCHOLOGIST

THE Clinical Psychologist spends most of her time in a psychiatric outpatient clinic practicing psychotherapy. She has devoted a great deal of time to the study of families of schizophrenic patients. She is thoroughly familiar with the uncertainties of the official classification scheme because she has found it frustratingly difficult to obtain homogeneous samples of schizophrenics for her research. She looks reflective and somewhat resigned to it all.

Inquirer: We are trying to improve the reliability of diagnostic categories. It seems that we have to reconsider our fundamental principles to develop a useful and defensible taxonomy.

Clinical
Psychologist: That seems clear to me also. Many psychologists are wary of the DSM-III system. They resist psychiatrists' notions that mental disorders represent a subset of medical diseases.[1] But this is in part a territorial interprofessional dispute. One seldom-mentioned objection to the official system is that it seems ridiculous in these times to try to invent names which not only label but purport to describe the disorder. "Schizophrenia" as a word means "split mind." What is a "split mind"? We should use neutral names for labels, such as Group II or Type B. You have more than problems of reliability to worry about. There are problems of validity, of specificity, and of coverage.

Inquirer: Validity is cited by everyone, from scientists to logicians to lawyers, as a good thing. What is your in-

---

[1]See Schacht, T., and Nathan, P. E.: But is it good for psychologists? Appraisal and status of DSM-III (*American Psychologist, 32*:1017, 1977). If disorders are defined according to the interventions used, then the largest part of medical practice is not literally medical but educational. Besides an occasional laying on of hands and injections, a physician mainly instructs the patient as to what he should do to and for himself to relieve his illness.

terpretation of the term?

Clinical
Psychologist: The term *validity* certainly has a bewildering number of uses. To a scientist, it can mean a *correct* theory; to a logician it can mean a *sound* argument; to a psychologist it can mean an *acceptable* construct. But then we also talk about the internal validity of test results (i.e. rerun consistency versus their external validity), meaning generalizability. In psychology, you will also hear of face validity, content validity, predictive validity, consensual validity, concurrent validity, construct validity and so forth.

Inquirer: Do all of these usefully apply to the domain of clinical problems?

Clinical
Psychologist: As has been noted, construct validity such as provided by an independent lab test would be fine. But under present conditions we would be doing well if we could stick to descriptive, concurrent, and predictive validities in trying to group patients. By "descriptive validity," I mean that the groups can be shown to be fairly homogeneous in respect to the properties shared by the members. By "concurrent validity," I mean that a variety of assessments — clinical observations, psychological tests, or measurements — lead to placing an individual in the same group. By "predictive validity," I mean one can predict the probable course of a disorder and its response to treatment. Practitioners are most interested in predictive utility. The clinical scientist is also interested in construct validity and the question of the cause of disorders. Causal factors, if they can be found, might be the strongest basis if not for treatment at least for prevention.[2]

---

[2]The deep causal waters have already been alluded to in the dialogue with the Biological Scientist. Causality as a philosophical concept seems straightforward enough. We interpret the expression P → Q to mean that P is a condition leading to, bringing about, producing or "causing" a condition Q. If whenever Q is found, P is found, then P is a necessary condition for

→

Inquirer:	You mentioned "specificity" as one of our problems.
Clinical Psychologist:	Many of the symptoms we use to place a patient in one category are found to occur in patients in other categories. For example, Schneider's first-rank symptoms, supposedly pathognomonic of schizophrenia, are also found in as high as 23 percent of manics. Much depends on your cutoff points. Suppose you have 100 cases of mental disorders. Using four symptoms, 80 of the cases might be identified as schizophrenic and 20 as belonging to other disorders. But if you require the patients to have 10 symptoms, only 20 will be identified as schizophrenia and *none* of the other disorders will show all 10 of the symptoms. Thus, the false positive ratio depends on the cutoff points.[3]
Inquirer:	So we lack specificity in that there are no properties *only* schizophrenics have. How about the "coverage" of a classification?
Clinical Psychologist:	By "coverage" I mean the percentage of patients who can be identified as members of the kinds in the classification scheme. When the rules for identifying patients as members of a kind are highly specific, many patients do not fit. If, as already mentioned, in order to be identified as "schizophrenic" you must be under 30 *and* unmarried *and* have delusions *and*

Q, that is, Q cannot occur without P. If, whenever P is found, Q is also found, the P is a sufficient condition for Q. Thus, if P were to occur, Q would occur. Sometimes P is both a necessary and sufficient condition for Q. We believe we have established a causal relation when we can produce Q by producing P. When we refrain from, or prevent, P, the Q does not occur. These manipulations tell us that P → Q relation is law-like and not an accidental generalization. In currently preferred jargon, P is called the independent variable and Q the dependent variable of this asymmetrical relation.

Now complexities appear in that both P and Q can represent multiple, compound conditions. Is the vulnerability of the host a cause of an infection? In medicine, some determinants are neither necessary nor sufficient. For example, in the association between low income and tuberculosis, we do not consider low income to be a "cause" but rather a contributory factor. The best strategy for psychiatry at the moment is to try to establish reliable and stable kinds which serve under Q and worry about the productive connection P → Q later.

[3]See Fenton, et al.: Diagnosis of schizophrenia (p. 412).

have hallucinations, those patients who lack this conjunction of properties will fall outside the kind "schizophrenia." Then what kind will they belong to? If all the kinds in the scheme are this tight and rigid, many patients will be unidentified because they fit no kind definition.

Statistical studies have shown that hypothetical, fictitious patients — those conceptualized as typical in the minds of psychiatrists — do fall into the traditional diagnostic categories.[4] But the great majority of *real* patients, both hospitalized and non-hospitalized, do not group into these categories. Real patients cluster in groups having low symptom scores with a greater heterogeneity of symptoms than diagnosticians realize. Some real patients do cluster in the traditional categories. These are patients with a few severe symptoms which stand out.[5]

It is known that human judgments are adversely affected by the process of "representativeness." That is, humans will judge the probability of X belonging to a kind by comparing X to a stereotype or prototype member of the kind. This leads them to neglect the sample size on which the prototype is based and to misestimate the prior probabilities, the base rates of the selected properties.[6] Accurate but unsystematic observations of such vivid "classical"

[4]See Overall, J. E., and Woodward, J. A.: Conceptual validity of a phenomenological classification of patients (*Journal of Psychiatric Research, 12*:214, 1975).

[5]Also, many clinicians believe symptoms are negatively correlated, whereas in real patients most symptoms are positively correlated. See Strauss, J. S., Gabriel, R., Kokes, R. F., Ritzler, B. A., Vanord, A. and Tarana, E.: Do psychiatric patients fit their diagnoses? Patterns of symptomatology as described with the biplot (*Journal of Nervous and Mental Disease, 167*:105, 1979).

[6]For some of our limitations as information processors and judges of people, see Tversky, A. and Kahneman, D.: Judgment under uncertainty: Heuristics and biases (*Science, 185*:1124, 1974), as well as Nisbett, R., and Ross, L.: *Human Inferences: Strategies and Shortcomings of Social Judgement* (New Jersey, Prentice Hall, 1980). For our peculiarities as logical reasoners, see Wason, P. C., and Johnson-Laird, P. N.: *Psychology of Reasoning: Structure and Content* (London, Batsford, 1965). When given increasing information, clinical judges use it simply to raise their confidence in the accuracy of their oft-mistaken decisions! See Goldberg, L. R.: Simple models or simple process? Some research in clinical judgements (*American Psychologist, 23*:483, 1968).

cases probably led clinicians of the past to form a classification system into which they tried to cram all patients. But the overemphasis put on a few distinctive or prominent symptoms resulted in a system with low coverage.

Inquirer: Why do you think clinicians cling to their encrusted classification system?

Clinical Psychologist: Current clinicians believe it because they have been taught to believe it. They don't have anything better to help them muddle through. A broken oar is better than no oar at all. Every once in a while they see a dramatic "classical" case and thereby have their beliefs in the stereotypes of the system reinforced. Coverage with our current scheme is poor at both ends. At one extreme, DSM-II had 100 percent coverage since it used wastebasket categories like "other." At the other extreme, the MMPI "cookbook" diagnosis has a coverage of only 25 percent.[7] We need to construct groups using a larger number of properties than we now have. You have heard it bluntly and simply put; we need new facts about patients.

Inquirer: Will psychological tests give us these facts?

Clinical Psychologist: That's a loaded question. Our track record with psychological tests has not been very impressive in the field of mental disorders. Many tests depended too much on clinicians' judgments for construction and validation. Take the MMPI. It was originally constructed in the late 1930s somewhat as follows. Patients diagnosed by psychiatrists were asked to answer *true* or *false* to 550 statements, and their responses were then compared to "normals'" responses. In constructing a particular scale, or dimension, diagnoses were used. For example, the hysteria scale was based on the responses given by patients diagnosed as "hysteric." But who deter-

[7]See Blashfield and Draguns, Toward a taxonomy of psychopathology (1976, p. 574).

mined the initial group had hysteria and how did they decide?

Inquirer: But once you get off the ground, can't you bootstrap it so that the scales become extended, predicting more than hysteria?

Clinical Psychologist: Yes, in fact the MMPI now predicts to conditions other than signs and symptoms, but its coverage of mental disorders is still far too low. Perhaps our most famous projective test, the Rorschach, turned out to be quite unreliable. Psychologists not only disagreed with one another about Rorschach data but two weeks later they didn't agree with their *own* judgments on the same original data. Both naive and clinical observers fail to recognize true co-variations or sign-symptoms association. Their judgments reflect a preconception of associations which "ought" to hold according to some handed-down or intuitive theory. Clinicians are extremely prone to report illusory correlations and, as to be expected, they are very confident in them.[8] I am all for objective tests, and I believe that the construction of such tests is necessary. But I don't have any handy at the moment.

Inquirer: As we have heard, every perception, observation, fact or measurement involves interpretation and judgment. The trick seems to be to gain intersubjective consensus by reducing arbitrary personal elements as much as possible. Is anyone working on devising new tests?

Clinical Psychologist: Some of my colleagues are. Many psychologists have become disenchanted with tests of mental disorders. Like myself, they have moved towards being therapists rather than testers. Psychologists

---

[8]See Chapman, L. J., and Chapman, J. P.: Illusory correlations as an obstacle to the use of valid diagnostic signs (*Journal of Abnormal Psychology, 74*:271, 1969). Like most human judges, once clinicians make up their mind about an association or correlation, it sticks there even in the face of counterevidence. Also, see Shneder, R.A.: Likeness and likelihood in everyday thought: Magical thinking in judgements about personality (*Current Anthropology, 18*:637, 1977).

who do psychotherapy research seem content with global outcome measures such as "improvement" or "ability to function" as judged by therapists, patients, or their relatives. This may be the best we can do for the time being. As the literature now indicates, such rough measures show that the condition of "neurotic" patients is 76 percent better than that of untreated controls assessed at the same time; that the benefits of treatment are stable for about one year and then gradually decline.[9] Psychotherapy is a coarsely defined set of interventions. We want to be able to apply specific therapeutic intervention to specific groups of patients rather than merely apply the vague kind "psychotherapy" to the vague kind "people with mental disorders." Such kinds are too crude to facilitate progress.

Inquirer:

We would not expect to formulate perfectly clear-cut and exact kinds of patients. The real world is a complex, fuzzy place and our brains are complex, sloppy systems, being made up mainly of water. How can anyone expect an organ made of water to have a perfect and exact representation of the world? As the Metaphysician instructs us, classes are human constructs. Their members cluster like swarms of bees with strays and outliers. A category like "schizophrenia" is very crude. But there are a few classical cases that fit the definitions.

Clinical
Psychologist:

In listening to what the Young Psychiatrist and Old Psychiatrist had to say about schizophrenia, another reason occurred to me why stubborn illusions about this disorder are perpetuated and why they are so hard to dispel. I attend weekly clinical case conferences in which patients

---

[9]See Smith, M. L., Glass, G. V., and Miller, T. I.: *The Benefits of Psychotherapy* (Baltimore, John Hopkins Press, 1980), as well as Andrews, G., and Harvey, R.: Does psychotherapy benefit neurotic patients? A reanalysis of the Smith, Glass, and Miller data (*Archives of General Psychiatry, 38*:1203, 1981). The main weakness of these studies and reviews is taxonomic since they lack data on diagnosis. What is a "neurotic" patient?

are discussed in detail.[10] Hardly a month goes by without the ritual invocation by some senior psychiatrist asserting that schizophrenics offer "concrete" interpretations of proverbs or that they follow the Von Domarus principle of making identifications on the basis of predicates rather than subjects. Yet both of these claims have been shown to be unfounded by numerous investigators who have demonstrated that no differences can be found between schizophrenics and normal controls when the groups are matched for educational level.[11]

Inquirer: What do they mean by "concrete"?

Clinical
Psychologist: Take proverbs. A psychiatrist will say to a patient, "A rolling stone gathers no moss — what does that mean to you?" The patient replies and then the psychiatrist decides on his own whether the response is literal, or concrete, or abstract, or whatever. Who is to say what is an abstract response? There are no agreed-on decision rules regarding the concrete-abstract dimensions. Thirty years ago there was no rock music group and no magazine called *Rolling Stone*. A senior psychiatrist today might get some interpretations of this proverb he would code as deviant but which are quite in keeping with the current musical scene.

Inquirer: Isn't there any characteristic of schizophrenia that has been found by tests?

Clinical
Psychologist: Kreitman and co-workers years ago reported zero percent agreement among five psychiatrists as to the presence of thought disorder.[12] The psychological and linguistic literature, however, indicates that

---

[10]For a devastating description of the intellectual banality of most of these case conferences, see Meehl, P.E.: Why I do not attend case conferences. In Meehl, P. E. (Ed.): *Psychodiagnosis: Selected Papers* (Minneapolis, University of Minnesota Press, 1973).

[11]See Williams, E. B.: Deductive reasoning in schizophrenia (*Journal of Abnormal and Social Psychology, 69*:47, 1964). Also Maher, B. A.: The Language of schizophrenia: A review and interpretation (*British Journal of Psychiatry, 120*:3, 1972).

[12]See Kreitman, et al.: Reliability of psychiatric assessment (p. 887).

there is something there, only it is difficult to pin down.

Inquirer: What do you mean there is something there?

Clinical
Psychologist: Several studies indicate that both clinicians and lay judges can discriminate "disordered" from "non-disordered" linguistic samples, both in written and spoken form, with an interjudge reliability of 0.7 and higher.[13] The clinicians do not do much better than undergraduates, but both can sort out the deviant linguistic products from the non-deviant. On what grounds they do it has not yet been clarified. But something we can designate as "deviant language" is present.

Inquirer: Do you mean undergraduates can distinguish schizophrenics from non-schizophrenics?

Clinical
Psychologist: Careful. I said linguistic samples. Some patients diagnosed as schizophrenic produce these deviant-language samples, whereas others do not. And not all linguistic output from the disordered schizophrenic group is judged deviant. In fact, most of their linguistic expressions are "normal." But every once in a while something appears which judges consider odd or deviant and take as an indicator of a disorder. One swallow does seem to make a summer in this case.

Inquirer: It would seem to me that you have a double taxonomic problem here. First, you must get agreements as to the kind *schizophrenia* and then you must get agreements regarding the kind

[13]This not-so-uncanny ability has been reported by Maher, B. A., McKean, K. O., and McLaughlin B.: Studies in psychotic language. In Stone, P. P., Dunphy, D. C., Smith, M. W., and Ogilvie, D. M. (Eds.): *The General Inquirer, A Computer Approach to Content Analysis* (Cambridge, MIT Press, 1966), as well as recently by Rochester, S. R., Martin, J. R., and Thurston, S.: Thought-process disorder in schizophrenia: The listener's task (*Brain and Language,* 4:95, 1977). For thorough reviews, see Rochester, S., and Martin, J. L.: *Crazy Talk, A Study of the Discourse of Schizophrenic Speakers* (New York, Plenum, 1979), and Schwartz, S.: *Language and Cognition in Schizophrenia* (Hillside, Erlbaum, 1978), as well as his, Is there a schizophrenic language? (*Behavioral and Brain Sciences,* 5:579, 1982). Another good article is Wykes, T.: Language and schizophrenia (*Psychological Medicine, 10*:403, 1980).

deviant language. To achieve this, you must have standards for *non-deviant* language. Once you have clarified the two kinds independently, the question becomes one of dyadic lawfulness. Can one make the law statement that whenever one has a member of the kind *schizophrenia*, one has a person whose language instantiates membership in the kind *deviant language* in some high percentage of cases? Notice that you cannot read the law statement backwards and claim that if someone shows deviant language, then he has schizophrenia.

Clinical
Psychologist: Why not? It would be saying that deviant language is one of the properties of schizophrenia.

Inquirer: You can get into a tautologous mess here. If you say deviant language is a property of schizophrenia, assign the label schizophrenia to people with deviant language and then study their linguistic expressions, you are going to unsurprisingly find some deviant language. The properties have to be delineated independently. People with pneumonia have fevers, but many other kinds of people have fevers also. From what you have said, the definitions of, and criteria for, deviant language are still unclear.

Clinical
Psychologist: Quite so. It is said that schizophrenics "say strange things." The statements pointed to are indeed strange to laymen and clinicians alike. As a clinician talking with patients, I have often been befuddled and baffled, finding them difficult to follow.[14]

---

[14]In information-theoretic terms, being "difficult to follow" is a property of the listener, not of the speaker. A listener selects from messages those features that are functionally important or salient to him. The meaning of a message is relative to an ensemble of alternatives whose ordering is determined by the recipient. See Dretske, Knowledge and the Flow of Information (p. 183). Experienced clinicians know that the longer one talks to a deviant-language patient and the more background information one obtains, the more the patient's expressions become less strange because it becomes clearer what he is referring to. This suggests such patients attribute to their first-time listeners too much information or too great a linguistic recognitional competence.

Inquirer:

Do you take the position that deviant language implies deviant thought or a thought disorder?

Clinical
Psychologist:

Much depends on how you regard the relation between language and thought. You might consider them identical, but most current opinion holds that they are two different processes operating under different rules. We take language expressions to be a vehicle for underlying ideational or thought processes. When a clinician or a lay judge notes something odd in a linguistic expression, what he observes is not a violation of a phonological or syntactical rule. If this were the case, the patient would have some sort of aphasia due to brain damage. The deviance of non-brain-damaged patients lies in the meaning or semantic area. The patient jumps around in utterances using submerged metaphors (cryptophors) so that it is hard, at times, to tell what he is referring to. The old clinicians called this behavior loose associations, derailments, cognitive slippage, or lack of coherence. If pressed for an explanation of his messages, however, the patient can usually clarify what he means in a way that makes sense.

Deviant language is not limited to patients called "schizophrenic." Peculiar speech has been found in other sorts of patients about as frequently as in schizophrenics.[15] Language deviance has been found in affective disorders, in normals who are fatigued, drunk, or talking in their sleep and in poetry by Dylan Thomas or E. E. Cummings.[16] There is something odd or bizarre about the thought processes of some patients as inferrable from

---

[15]See Andreason, N. C., and Grove, W.: The relationship between schizophrenic language, manic language, and aphasia. In Gauzelier, J. and Flor-Henry, P. (Eds.): *Hemisphere Assymetries of Function In Psychopathology* (Amsterdam, Elsevier/North Holland, 1979).

[16]See Reed, J. L.: Schizophrenic thought disorder: A review and hypothesis (*Comprehensive Psychiatry, 11*:403, 1970), as well as Harrow, M., and Quinlan, D.: Is disordered thinking unique to schizophrenia? (*Archives of General Psychiatry, 34*:15, 1977).

their odd linguistic expressions. But we still have no systematic way of distinguishing instances of thought disorders from non-instances. The problem is how to characterize them further.

Inquirer: Wasn't it shown that even the parents of schizo- phrenics produced more deviant speech than the parents of neurotics?

Clinical
Psychologist: The original study has not been replicated by others. It may be that the parents of schizophrenics simply talk more. From my own work with families of "schizophrenics," I can see why they would have a lot more to talk about.[17]

Inquirer: Given the evidence you present, how do you ac- count for the fact that psychiatrists, at least until the recent publication of DSM-III, still used proverb interpretations and "thought disorder" to diagnose schizophrenia?

Clinical
Psychologist: My only explanation is that psychiatrists, especially once they get into practice, do not read the literature and especially not the research literature. Then when they run or attend a case conference, they simply repeat what was told them when they were residents. The young psychiatrists believe what the experienced clinician says, and so the mythical correlations about schizophrenia go on and on.

Inquirer: Why don't you speak up about it at these case con- ferences?

Clinical
Psychologist: I did for awhile, but who is going to listen to a wom- an psychologist flying in the face of overwhelming medical authority. Anyway, this part of psychia- trists' act has been partly cleaned up by DSM-III, which as you have pointed out on many occasions,

---

[17]The original study was Singer, M. T., and Wynne, L. C.: Communication styles in parents of normals, neurotics, and schizophrenics (*Psychiatric Research Reports, 20*:25, 1966). The "talk- ing more" hypothesis comes from Hirsch, S. R., and Leff, J. R.: *Abnormalities in Parents of Schizophrenics* (London, Oxford University Press, 1975).

has it own problems.

Inquirer: The behavior modification psychologists have not seemed reluctant to challenge psychiatric authority.

Clinical
Psychologist: But only in the area of treatment. For reasons I do not understand, they have swallowed whole the official psychiatric classification scheme. There are many reports on the behavior modification of schizophrenia, simply taking for granted that schizophrenia is a reliable category that one can use in determining the effectiveness of behavior therapy. If psychiatrists say a patient has schizophrenia, many psychologists naively accept it. Notice that psychologists also adopted the official scheme and even proposed causes for such things as "hysteria." The clinical field has not seemed to be able to grasp that there is a basic problem here. If you go long enough not thinking something is wrong, you begin to think it might be right.

Inquirer: The Old Psychiatrist says psychology should be to psychiatry as physiology is to medicine. That is, psychology should first provide us with a taxonomy of normal mental functions. Then we can say what mental disorder is because we know what the normal range of values is for mental functions. We would have an order to compare to disorder.

Clinical
Psychologist: I can see the virtue of this analogy, but it is not as easy to say what a normal value of a mental function is as it is to say what a normal pulse rate is. The pulse rate involves a direct observation on which one can gain consensus easily. Some overt human behavior, such as handwashing hundreds of times a day, is obviously abnormal. But what about uninspectable covert behaviors such as thoughts, fantasies, affects and beliefs? The main products of mental activity in consciousness are fantasies. What is a normal fantasy? What is a normal belief? What is a normal idea?

Inquirer: Surely, someone nowadays who believes, and says, that he is Jesus Christ is suffering from a disorder.

Clinical
Psychologist: The blatant cases are easy. Delusions of persecution or grandeur are obvious cases when they are expressed in language or in overt behavior. It is getting at what is "inside" the mind, the uninspectables, and judging them to represent disorder that is so difficult because many inferences have to be made to connect overt behavior with covert internal patterns and processes. There has even been a long and strong tradition in psychology that the mind was not a respectable focus of inquiry. Only overt behavior was to be considered worthy of a science. In this respect, strict behaviorism was not just an evasion but also a bad idea. Today, clinical psychology is disillusioned. It has not delivered the goods, at least in advancing knowledge about mental disorders. It has been too simplistic about a complex subject matter. As my colleague, the Mind Scientist, indicated, there is now a great revival of interest in the mental under the name of the "cognitive sciences."[18] If you want to know more about scientific aspects of mental disorders, you should talk to the Psychiatric Scientist.

Inquirer: I hear he wants to have a say.

---

[18]See Fodor, *Representations*, and Simon, H.: Cognitive science: the newest science of the artificial (*Cognitive Science, 4*:33, 1980).

Dialogue VIII

THE PSYCHIATRIC SCIENTIST

T HIS Psychiatric Scientist, somewhat out of step with the biochemical times, views mental disorders mainly from a mental-
level perspective. His research traditions are those of medicine,
psychodynamic psychiatry, and cognitive psychology. Now his interest is in the cognitive sciences. He views the field through the lens
of a computer metaphor and constantly refers to this infernal semantic engine, which is most annoying to those who neither understand,
nor want to understand, how the contraption works.

Inquirer: We are trying to improve the diagnostic classification
scheme in psychiatry, and the Clinical Psychologist
suggested I talk with you.

Psychiatric
Scientist: One aspect of the official scheme has not yet been
touched on in your dialogues and that is the logic, or
lack of it, in psychiatric classification. Much like the
ninth century Chinese classification you heard about
from the Biological Scientist, the diagnostic system
lacks a uniform taxonomic principle by which patients
can be grouped. It lacks a *fundamentum divisionis* — an
ordering principle for dividing things up. Some
disorders are classified according to symptoms, some
according to behaviors, some according to postulated
etiologies. It's as if you had a collection of hats and
then grouped them into brown hats, round hats, rain
hats, tall hats, felt hats, hard hats, and so on. It's a
mess. As John Dunne would say, "'Tis all in peeces, all
cohaerance gone."

Inquirer: That seems agreed on by most of us. The Clinicial
Psychologist suggested I talk to you about the concepts of mental disorder and disease. Maybe
psychiatric patients should not be viewed as having
diseases.

132

Psychiatric
Scientist: The books tell us that Thomas Sydenham in the seventeenth century proposed that there were species of disease, which he considered to be natural kinds, just as there were biological species.[1] He had a concept of a cluster or syndrome. He thought the cluster should be named, not only in accordance with its present manifestations, but also according to its evolving course, its natural history. Syndenham's analogy between disease and species cannot be carried too far. One can be a member of only a single species but one can be a member of several classes of disease simultaneously.

In the subsequent 300 years, the concept of physical diseases and their taxonomy, called *nosology*, has added further elements. Today, a medical textbook definition would state a disease involves: (a) etiological agents or causes, (b) a pathogenesis which represents the body's reaction to etiological events, (c) morphological, functional, chemical, etc. changes which result in producing (d) signs and symptoms in the patient. The big question for us in psychiatry is whether some, or any, of these conceptual elements of physical disease apply to mental disorders.

Inquirer: If this definition works in medicine, why don't you adopt it in psychiatry?

Psychiatric
Scientist: Mainly because we don't know enough to fill in the (a), (b), and (c) components of the definition. Nor does medicine always approximate this ideal definition. For example, except for infections and intoxications, the causes of most diseases are unknown. Disease is a useful concept when one knows its cause; otherwise it is of doubtful value.[2] It is usually more valuable to the clinician to know about the underlying mechanisms involved in the illness process. Once these are discovered, a clinical

---

[1]Feinstein, *Clinical Judgment* (p. 104).
[2]See Scadding, J. G.: The romantics of medical diagnosis (*International Journal of Biomedical Computing*, 3:83, 1972), as well as Kendell, R. E., *Role of Diagnosis in Psychiatry*.

taxonomy can improve, being based now, not on the manifest properties typical of a Sydenham cluster, but on the anomalies found in the underlying mechanisms. Thus, a viral pneumonia is managed differently from a pneumococcal pneumonia. Let me show you some of the intricate causal relations touched on in your talk with the Biological Scientist.[3] Notice the complexities that are possible with only a few variables.

Scadding, a British expert on medical diagnosis, defines disease as "the sum of the abnormal phenomena displayed by a group of living organisms in association with a specified common characteristic or set of characteristics by which they differ from the norm for their species in such a way as to place them at a biological disadvantage."[4] The irrelevance of this definition for psychiatry is that few of our patients show a biological disadvantage in terms of mortality or fertility rates. There is more to human life than survival and breeding.

Inquirer: Didn't medical diagnosis improve by using further statistical and mathematical aids, and why couldn't psychiatry do the same?

Psychiatric
Scientist: It was mainly through better laboratory tests and controlled experiments that medicine has progressed. Mathematical aids to diagnostic reasoning have been limited. The logic or lines of reasoning a medical diagnostician uses is still not well understood.[5] Attempts have been made to improve these expert judgments using a relative frequency form of conditional-probability theory.[6] Given the evidence E

[3]He draws diagrams of Figure 4 on the blackboard and labels the relations using specific medical examples. See Susser, M.: *Causal Thinking in the Health Sciences* (New York, Oxford) for a discussion of causality more complex than the philosopher's necessary and sufficient conditions.

[4]See Scadding, J. G.: Diagnosis: the clinician and the computer (*Lancet* 2:877, 1967).

[5]See Feinstein, A., Englehardt, H.T., Spicker, S.F., and Towers, B. (Eds.): *Clinical Judgement*: A Critical Appraisal (Hingham, Reidel, 1979).

[6]See Murphy, E. A.: *Probability in Medicine* (Baltimore, Johns Hopkins University Press, 1979).

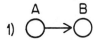

Example: Streptococcus causes pneumonia.

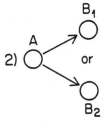

Example: Streptococcus causes pneumonia or
meningitis.

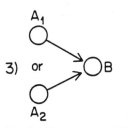

Example: Streptococcus or pneumococcus
causes pneumonia.

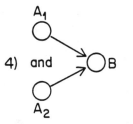

Example: Defective enzyme and diet containing phenylalanine causes phenylke-
tonuria.

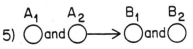

Example: Defective enzyme and diet containing phenylalanine causes multiple
effects on head size and intelligence.

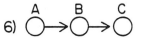

Example: Sickle cell anemia causes brain
damage which causes paralysis.

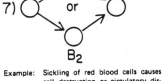

Example: Sickling of red blood cells causes
cell destruction or circulatory dis-
turbances which cause heart failure.

Figure 4. (A = cause, B = effect, → = causes, produces, brings about)

about a patient, what is the probability P that he has
disease D? That is, P(D/E)? And when a patient has
disease D, what is the probability that some evidence
E can be found regarding him, i.e. P(E/D)? And what
is the probability of D and E, in the sense of relative
frequency, in the population? Which population —
the population at large, the patient population, the
hospitalized population?

In a few medical conditions, this approach has seemed promising, but most of the time the actual numbers for the probability values, the quantitative data, are not available.[7]

A straight probability gives an estimate of a single event, such as the probability of Borg winning Wimbledon next year is 0.33, or in terms of odds, if Borg were to play Wimbledon three times, he would win it once. A conditional probability concerns two events and estimates the probability of one given the other. Thus, given that a patient has symptoms S_1, what is the probability that he has disorder D_1 i.e. $P(D_1/S_1)$? The simplest formal version for a disorder D with evidence E is:

$$P(D/E) = \frac{P(E/D \times P)}{P(E)}$$

Modifications have been made in the denominator, but they need not concern us here. The big problem for us is that we do not know precisely the frequency of a disease in the population at large, or the frequency of the evidence in a given disease, or the frequency of the evidence in the patient population. The numerator of the relative frequencies is taken usually from hospitalized cases and the denominator from the census. Because these data are imprecise currently does not mean they could not be improved. Even if we knew these numbers, would it help medical diagnosis? In psychiatry, the whole problem can be ignored for the time being until we obtain a firmer and more reliable grasp of what the D's and E's are.

Inquirer: Do diagnostic experts think in terms of relative frequency probabilities?

---

[7]They are getting into the haze of Bayes and his theorem for conditional probabilities. For a thorough treatment of Bayes' theorem in medicine, see Feinstein, A. R., Clinical biostatistics XXXIX: The haze of Bayes, the aerial palaces of decision analysis and the computerized Ouija board (*Clinical Pharmacology and Therapeutics*, 21:482-496, 1977); also, cf. Galen, R. S., and Gambino, S. R., *Beyond Normality*, and Nozick , R.: *Philosophical Explanations* (Cambridge, Harvard University Press, 1981, p. 254-261).

Psychiatric
Scientist: Probably not, or at least not with any exact knowledge
of frequency rates. They have beliefs about diseases
which do not follow the axioms of conventional probability theory. For example, probability theory would
say that if P(D/E) is 0.7, the probability of *not* having
D should be 0.3 since these probabilities must add up
to 1 in a classical probability calculus. But diagnosticians do not trust the usefulness of this mathematical
view when it is applied to clinical conditions. They
claim that the same evidence for D should not also
favor the absence of D. For example, if a 60-year-old
male cigarette smoker is coughing blood, has lost
weight, and has a pulmonary shadow on X-ray, a
clinician might be willing to say the patient has lung
cancer with a probability of 0.9. But he would not
agree this evidence denies lung cancer with a probability of 0.1. He would say the evidence, thus far, for
the denial of lung cancer should be zero, and I agree
with him. Evidence for denial would be a biopsy
showing the pulmonary lesion to be a benign tumor.

Inquirer: This may be the way diagnosticians think, but maybe
this is not the way they *should* think. There is a
descriptive and a normative perspective here.

Psychiatric
Scientist: Negations and denials can be ambiguous.[8] Say you
do not believe (B) in some proposition (P). Does this
mean not belief in P, i.e. ¬B(P) or does it mean belief
in not P, i.e. B(¬P)? The hesitant confession of wrongdoing is different from the confession of hesitant
wrongdoing. No expert diagnostician is going to
let pure relative frequencies dominate his diagnostic
decisions. He wants to rule out plausible candidates
for the disease regardless of their frequency. He com-
bines inclusion and exclusion with the rival-candidate
set.[9]

---

[8]There are no negative properties in the world. For example, "non-blue" is not a color. Negation is a conceptual-cognitive operation we utilize for human purposes.

[9]The Psychiatric Scientist is perhaps ennobling the clinician here. In their own minds, clini-
→

Inquirer: The diagnostician is relying on his beliefs, his personal credibility functions, more than probability functions. But then how do we know his beliefs are correct or justifiable?

Psychiatric
Scientist: Here is where you would have to have some sort of systematic learning system in which the starting credibilities of experts are modified by feedback from the actual outcomes in patients. Such records would even give you the probability of the evidence given the disease (P(E/D)), which is now mainly unknown. All we can find in our current handwritten records are numerators.[10] We need denominators as well to get standards of comparison for abnormality or distinctiveness.

Inquirer: I gather, then, that you don't think the general analogy with medical diagnosis in physical conditions will be very fruitful in psychiatry dealing with mental conditions.

Psychiatric
Scientist: It would be easy to say "no," but there are a number of worthwhile analogies. Diagnoses involve human judgments. Humans have both information-processing abilities and limitations. In ·probability

---

cians do use crude probabilities, in the sense of frequency ratios, without realizing it. There is an old maxim in medicine — "When you hear hoofbeats think of horses, not zebras." This is a conditional probability of the form P (horses/hooves) (i.e. the probability of horses, given hearing hoofbeats).

It is a subjective probability representing a degree of personal belief. Notice the negation again. There is a difference between not thinking of zebras and thinking it is not zebras. Also, the setting is important. In Boston, you might not think of zebras, but on the Serengeti Plain in Africa, you would think not only of zebras but even of wildebeests.

[10]Machine-readable records are patient records that a computer can rapidly scan through looking for desired information. Most current psychiatric records are a hopeless mess, combining handwritten notes, whose illegibility is directly proportional to the hostility of the interns and residents forced to write them, and typewritten summaries giving diagnostic conclusions but not the evidence. Searching for specific data in past records "by hand" is time-consuming and frustrating since there are no fixed positions in the records where the data can be found (sometimes they are in the nurses' notes). Suppose you wanted to find out how many Mexican-American women, admitted to the hospital over the past three years, had a diagnosis of schizophrenia and were left-handed. Manually, it would take weeks or months. If the records were in a machine-readable form, the task could be performed in a few minutes. Psychiatry resists high technology.

judgments, they tend to be conservative, truncating at both high and low ends of a probability scale. Diagnosticians usually consider only six to eight alternatives. Above eight items, their performance decreases even though more information is being supplied.[11] You heard from the Clinicial Psychologist about the perils of the "representativeness" problem in which an individual is compared to a stereotype member of a class. Humans also tend to estimate the probability of an event from their ease of recall. Thus, vividness of examples, efficiency of search, and goodness of memory are factors. Finally, there exist anchorings in which an estimate is biased by the starting point.[12] All these limitations apply to psychiatric as well as medical diagnoses.

Inquirer: Is there any significant way in which a medical diagnosis of physical disorders differs from a psychiatric diagnosis of mental disorders?

Psychiatric
Scientist: First, let's back up and clarify some points about the mental and the physical, then we can get to the disorders these adjectives might apply to. I am an unabashed mentalist in the Mind Scientist's sense. I believe it is realistic and fruitful to conceive that people have an internal representational model of their experience that is partly responsible for those overt observable behaviors of a person we call courses of action. I contrast informed courses of action to mere movements. Without getting enmired in the mind-brain problem, I make the assumption that traditional mental entities, described in ordinary terms as *desires*, *affects*, *beliefs*, and *intentions* have some ultimate connection with the functioning of brain cells. Descartes did not get it quite right. We are not made up of two substances, mental and physical, but of one "substance"

---

[11]See Jacquez, J. A., and Norusis, M. J.: The importance of symptom non-independence in diagnosis. In DeDombal and Grenay (Eds.), *Decision Making and Medical Care. For how few alternatives we can keep in consciousness at a given time*, see Simon, H.: How big is a chunk? *(Science, 183*:482, 1974).

[12]See Tversky and Kahneman, Judgment under uncertainty (1974, p. 1125).

(if you want to call information a substance) that is capable of being in a variety of states or phases. At the level of person language, we have numerically one entity (i.e. the person as agent that can be viewed prismatically from a plurality of aspects). A person level of explanation would use intentional terms of natural language describing a person's wants, beliefs, purposes, plans, etc. At the subpersonal level of a person's parts and processes, the natural language terms become "denaturalized" referring, for example, to patterned data structures as belief analogues.[13]

The clearest example of a mental/physical system is a computer system. It is numerically one symbol-matter information-processing system, but its behavior can be analyzed from the perspective of its physical hardware or from the perspective of the program that the hardware is running. The biperspectival view allows us to have two means of access, two modes of knowing and talking about one thing. The numerically single computational system is simultaneously under dual controls of hardware and program. The program is dependent upon the hardware, but the behavior of the hardware is governed by the program. In linguistic terms, the duality is one of sense but not of reference. The physical behavior of the hardware abides by or obeys the semantic relations encoded in the symbols and rules of the program. If the system does not behave the way it is supposed to, a search begins for the reason. If it is a hardware failure, a wire or chip may have to be replaced. If there is an error in the program, the program must be corrected. You don't fix a program error with a screwdriver.

Inquirer: I foresee you are going to claim there is an analogy between physical and mental disease by bludgeoning

---

[13]There is no need to abandon the terms of everyday folk psychology. Physics took the everyday term *force* and added the technical meaning as the rate of change of momentum. Current particle physics speaks of *nakedness, charm,* and *strangeness*. Science progresses not only by successive approximations but by successive redefinitions of its concepts. We can define *belief* in a technical way as a type of representation, a data structure, having a property of truth-value. The advantage is a gain in explicitness and, if necessary, the belief structure can be drawn on a blackboard and ostensively pointed to.

us with computer analogies.[14]

Psychiatric
Scientist: Until the invention of the computer, this whole prob-
                    lem was difficult to get straight, or even to think about
                    easily, because we lacked an object in the real world,
                    besides ourselves, that exemplified how the mental
                    and the physical could be sensibly related.[15] I will try
                    to persuade you that there is a fruitful analogy be-
                    tween mental and physical *disorder*, not disease, and
                    that this analogy is exemplified by disorders in com-
                    putational systems.

Inquirer: You first have to *dis*suade me from the notion that
                    mental disorders are not physical disorders since you
                    admit the entities of the mental level correlate with the
                    functioning of neurons.

Psychiatric
Scientist: You went through some of this with the Mind Scien-
                    tist. I will take it further. The reason we need to posit
                    a representational system or internal model which is
                    symbolically rather than neuron defined is that there
                    exists no necessary exact correspondence between
                    structure and function in a computer. By this, I mean
                    that the same addresses or physical locations in a com-
                    puter can be used for a great variety of program func-
                    tions. At one moment a given location will be used by
                    a chess-playing program deciding on its next move,
                    and at another moment this same location in this same
                    machine will be engaged in finding a word-synonym

---

[14]It is curious how man often thinks of himself in terms of his own artifacts. The heart is viewed as a pump and muscle control is compared to power steering. Wilson compares mental
disorder to a poorly tuned auto engine in which there is nothing wrong with the engine's constitutive parts but their functions are not properly synchronized or coordinated, resulting in a
malfunctioning or maladjusted system. See Wilson *Mental as Physical* (pp. 334-336). Such
analogies can make objects and processes more accessible to analysis.

[15]It was no accident that computers were invented in a mental image of ourselves. Humans may not be machines, but parts of them behave *like* some machines. The heart behaves
like a pump and our minds behave like some computer programs. If we must be consoled,
we can say our minds are like *very special kinds* of machines and not just like any old machine
like a steam shovel or an electric can opener. Minds and brains are homologous, whereas
models of the mind are analogous. If it could be constructed, a formal computational structure of mind would be *theoretically* identical with the formal computational structure of the
brain.

in a language-recognition program.[16] Not only is this true for a given computer but it holds for other computers of the same brand and of the same design.

In human brains, there is no necessary correspondence between physical location and function, except in some very gross senses, like the occipital lobe involves vision and Broca's area involves speech. Hence, we must make room for the view that there can be a disorder of mental function not consistently involving any particular point-specific physical location or, in our case, any particular set of neurons in concert.

Inquirer: But no matter where they are exactly, neurons are involved, and neurons are physical things vulnerable to physical disorders.

Psychiatric
Scientist: Of course. It is not that neurons are irrelevant, but knowledge about neurons is irrelevant for working out the properties and laws of the symbolic-computational layers in that big jump between synapse and sentence. Neurons are incessantly at work.[17] But that does not imply that mental disorders are definable in terms of specific, fine-grained anatomical structures such as

---

[16]If we compare neurons with computer addresses, there are a few important disanalogies. Neurons die and disappear, some say at the rate of 100,000 per day, others say at the rate of one per mintue. When a neuron dies, another neuron may substitute for it. A neuron that at time t_1 particpated in a given firing pattern may not do so at time t_2 because (a) it is in its refractory period with its resting potential building after the last action potential discharge, (b) it is currently engaged in some other firing pattern, and (c) it is in an inhibited state produced by transmitters from other neurons. How all this is organized and coordinated is, thankfully, a problem for neural scientists.

[17]The neurophysiologist Mountcastle has provided a picturesque description of ourselves and the plight of our neurons: "Each of us believes himself to live directly within the world that surrounds him, to sense its objects and events precisely, to live in real and current time. I assert these are perceptual illusions, for each of us confronts the world from a brain linked to 'what is out there' by a few million fragile sensory fibers. These are our only information channels, our lifelines to reality. These sensory fibers are not high fidelity recorders, for they accentuate certain stimulus features, neglect others. The *central neuron is a story-teller* with regard to the afferent nerve fibers; and he is never completely trustworthy, allowing distortions of quality and measure, within a strained but isomorphic spatial relation between 'inside' and 'outside.' Sensation is an abstraction, not a replication, of the real world" (italics added). See Mountcastle, V. B.: The view from within: pathways to the study of perception (*Johns Hopkins Medical Journal, 136*:109, 1975).

cell-assemblies. Remember the hardware-program distinction and the dual controls of a computer system. In a program disorder, it is the program, embodied in some hardware location, that is causing the hardware components of other locations to operate in a way they are not supposed to. The program is the ghost in the machine which has spooked some philosophers.[18] Popper and Eccles, being surprisingly naive about computers, even state there must exist a homunculus in the brain playing on the neurons the way a person plays a piano. This is ghostly interactionist dualism galore.[19]

Inquirer: But computer people talk as if there was a little man in the machine. They use all kinds of anthropomorphic terms in describing the system as seeing, deciding, thinking, etc. They say a chess-playing program is "thinking about its next move."

Psychiatric Scientist: It is because this is an efficient way of communicating in high-level descriptions. Ordinary language is more abstract than realized. One could describe what is happening in the system in terms of millions of on-off switches and bit-patterns, but it would take a long time.[20] Here is an example where the detailed description could be correct but overly intractable. Convenience for communication as well as correctness is a desideratum for descriptions and explanations. The program is not a homunculus, but, in a way, its func-

---

[18]See Ryle, G.: *The Concept of Mind* (London, B & N, 1949).

[19]See Popper, K. R., and Eccles, J. C.: *The Self and Its Brain* (New York, Springer, 1977). The piano analogy is apposite for anyone who knows how a player piano works. Paper rolls with holes generate the music when a roll is turned; no homunculus is required since the rolls can be turned electrically as well as by a human pumping the pedals. Computer illiteracy should become increasingly infrequent in future mind-brain debates.

[20]The motions of a grandfather and his grandson on a see-saw could be described in terms of quantum mechanics, but the description would be a bit unwieldy, involving thousands of equations requiring several million years to solve. Who would bother to check them all out? A description of the see-saw motions in classical mechanics involving the principle of a lever is much more serviceable, expedient, and provides a satisficing approximation. *Exact* truth requires exact measurements which in turn require an infinite amount of energy. Hence, scientists must be satisfied with approximations.

tional parts and processes could be described as a coalition of progressively simpler homunculi with each having a specific procedure to carry out. As you go farther and farther down in the system, the homunculi become less and less clever, finally saying in effect only "yes" or "no." The lowest homunculus is a wire, which when charged with five volts means "yes" and zero volts means "no." To many people, it is uncanny that such a system with only varying voltages at the bottom can defeat them at chess. But it is no more mysterious than a system of neurons that fire or do not fire. How could *that* system ever play chess?

Inquirer: You said you wanted to discuss disorder, not disease. If you are going to use an analogy with physical disease, why not continue with the concept of disease at the mental level?

Psychiatric
Scientist: An analogy involves comparing two things. The positive analogy represents properties they share, the negative analogy represents properties they do not share, and a neutral zone represents properties whose positive or negative status we can't yet decide about. I want to say there is a positive analogy between mental disorders and physical disease to the extent they both represent something being wrong with the system. But now I want to separate the mental from the physical and point to the negative analogy of something wrong with the hardware versus something wrong with the program. Because of the hardware-program distinction, the concept of dual control and the lack of exact structure-function correspondence, I believe it is tenable to propose a relatively autonomous area of certain, not all, mental disorders. It isn't that mental representations are completely autonomous, but that they are neutral to their physical realizations or embodiments. A mental disorder can be viewed as a symbolic-program disorder and treated by reprogramming through a high-level language such as natural language as well as by other methods.

Inquirer: As a crude and purely physical input, suppose I pound on the hardware with a hammer hard enough to damage it. Can't I produce observable pathological behavior or malfunction in a computer that is indistinguishable from that produced by a disordered program?

Psychiatric
Scientist: In principle, yes, and perhaps some disorders that we now call mental will turn out to have a purely physical, non-symbolic cause of this nature. But the "pounding" performed will have to be quite sophisticated and microscopically specific. Recall my argument about the lack of a finely grained structure-function correspondence. If you damage one location, you will produce a malfunction because of an interference with the program being run at that moment using that location. But when the program is run again, it may use other locations and no malfunction will result, at least from that program. However, other programs that become assigned to the damaged location will not function properly, and now you will observe a great variety of malfunctions appearing.

You might offer, as a counterexample, linguistic functions which we know are carried out by a rather restricted area of the brain. Metaphorically, pounding in that area produces a variety of aphasias. But I doubt if you could pound those cells which assign gender to Italian nouns in such a way that the person consistently will utter the mistaken "il mano" instead of the correct "la mano." American tourists make this mistake because they follow the Italian language rule "nouns ending in 'o' are masculine." To correct this error, the tourist must be supplied correct information to reprogram himself at a cognitively penetrable level. The fine structure of the program does not correspond to the fine structure of anatomy. If you want to interfere with a specific function in a specific program that can be run in alternative areas of the system, you would have to pound away at, and damage, the system so extensively that you would get absolutely chaotic disorder in almost all of its functions.

Sydenham has a point about syndromes. Disorders are not chaotic; they are like species or natural kinds, clusters possessing law-like patterns and properties. They have norms of their own. When a highly ordered and structured system is perturbed, it reacts in an orderly way unless it completely disintegrates. Mental disorders represent perturbations and interferences in computational functions.

Inquirer: So let's say there can be mental disorders that are physico-symbolic, involving symbols in a medium, and view them as computational dysfunctions. How do you identify a mental *dis*-order?

Psychiatric
Scientist: A couple of times I have slipped in phrases such as "the way it is supposed to," hoping that I would be caught out. To say that something represents a dysfunction, one must first be able to determine what standard or proper functioning is. Scholarly psychiatrists realize we lack a theory of mental disorder. It's worse than that. We lack a theory of mental order, a proper working order indicating a well-functioning system. What is a well-functioning system? It is one that is in proper working order according to specified rules of right-functioning; one that is doing what it is supposed to do, what it is *designed* to do.

Inquirer: How do you know what a system is designed to do? And who designed it?

Psychiatric
Scientist: Please, one deep and dark question at a time. As has been brought up in the previous dialogues, two sorts of interrelatable systems are involved here: a theoretical system and its application to empirical systems. Let me rehearse the argument because it is an extremely important one to understand.

One constructs, conjectures, and hypothesizes an idealized kind of system described in a set of stipulated definitions. The deliberately idealized system is a woven web of guesses, aloof from all the details of its empirical counterparts, but having one or more empirical system in mind during its formulation. As our venerable example, Newton constructed a theoretical system of bodies or particles in motion using what he called *laws* and what we would today call *definitions*. The definitions specify the design of the system. His first law stated that a body remains at rest or in motion unless a force acts on it. Thus, it represents an idealized system because we know that in empirical systems all bodies have forces acting on them. Now the question is, what kinds of empirical systems might satisfy the definitions of the postulated system. Several or one or none might approximate it. For 300 years people took the empirically observable solar system as satisfying the definitions of a Newtonian particle system even though it (especially the perihelion of Mercury) did not quite fit demands of the ideal system. In the twentieth century, people came to believe the solar system better satisfied the definitions of an Einsteinian particle system. Even this improvement was not entirely satisfactory because the only forces involved were gravitational, omitting all the other forces, such as electromagnetic, that we know are active in the real solar system. When optical phenomena did not fit very well with a Newtonian particle system, it was not concluded that the system was false, but simply that light did not consist of particles. Newton's theoretical system could handle a sun-earth or a moon-earth empirical system, but it failed to handle a sun-moon-earth system (the three-body problem). The theoretical system is not false; it just does not apply, its scope is limited.

Inquirer: You have lost me. What does all this have to do with our problem?

Psychiatric
Scientist: One should never use examples from the history of physics. My point is we need to postulate a theory of

the design of an optimal, well-functoning mental system. Then we investigate empirical mental systems to see how well they satisfy or approximate the specifications of the ideal design. When they do not, we may have a mental disorder by definition, or we may lack sufficient knowledge of the empirical system, or we may have a poor theoretical system to start with. You can find out what an empirical system is designed to do by studying it. One can look at all of biology as a problem in design analysis. What is the design of organisms, and what is the source of this design?[21] Biologists seem to agree that organisms are systems whose designs keep themselves going and reproduce themselves. The source of this design is supposed to be an evolutionary process regulated by variation and natural selection.

Inquirer: The design problem in the study of mental activity is how to specify the structure of a theoretic and idealized symbolic-representational system and to specify how it optimally functions when in proper working order. What would the theory for a representational system in humans state the mental system is designed to do?

Psychiatric
Scientist: What makes the computer analogy a powerful one, at least to some of us, is that brains and computers are physical sytems, using symbolic languages and codes, that are able successfully to solve problems of intelligence-requiring tasks. We want to understand the design of the empirical mental systems of persons. The ideal design does not insist on any particular physical realization, but the evolutionary fact that it has been achieved by the human brain must be significant. The AI (artificial intelligence) brotherhood tends to evade this biological fact.[22]

---

[21]It is interesting that neural scientists, when they look at the anatomy of a ganglion, a tract, or a neuron, say to themselves, "I wonder what it *does*, what is it *for*?" (personal communications from neural colleagues). Without saying so, they are asking design questions.

[22]One cannot do everything at once. Certain problems must be finessed so that others can be worked on. AI bypasses a lot more than evolutionary fact. It ignores consciousness and the human brain, shrugging off the hardware fact that the brain is 80 percent water and runs on 15 watts! See Pattee, H.H.: Cell psychology: An evolutionary approach to the symbol-matter problem (*Cognition and Brain Theory*, 5:325, 1982) as well as Newell, A.: Physical symbol systems (*Cognitive Science*, 4:135, 1980).

If we can say what the postulated mental system is supposed to do and compare it to empirical systems, then we can say an empirical system does or does not satisfy the specification standards of working properly to an acceptable degree of approximation. The empirical data are adjusted back to the standards of the ideal system that serves as a heuristic or epistemic aid without necessary ontological status. Wasn't it the Old Psychiatrist who said psychology should be to psychiatry as physiology is to medicine? If we turn to psychology for help in our design analysis, we find a curious state of affairs, as the Clinical Psychologist pointed out. Many psychologists have been interested purely in overt behavior rather than in what generates that behavior.[23] The design problem should be the province and delight of psychology.

Inquirer: Isn't psychology defined as the science of human behavior rather than of mental capacities?

Psychiatric
Scientist: It depends on what you mean by behavior. The behavior of what and under what description? Everything can be said to behave. In humans you probably don't mean reflex behavior, but, instead, external informed and rational actions. If you limit your concern to the overt actions of persons, snags appear when it comes to deciding what is proper functioning and what is not. Focusing solely on external action makes us highly susceptible to confounding social deviance with mental disorder. Such judgments of manifest behavior are dependent upon what a culture or social system holds to be right or wrong.

In a dry town in the Midwest, a man who drinks a few beers a week may be considered an alcoholic. A

---

[23]One does not explain behavior by behavior. One theoretically explains temperature as the kinetic energy of molecules which themselves do not have a temperature. Confusion of *explanadum* with the *explanans* is common in the behavioral sciences. The definitive demolition of behaviorism can be found in Chomsky, N.: A review of B. F. Skinner's *Verbal Behavior*. Reprinted in Fodor, J. A., and Katz, J. J. (Eds.): *The Structure of Language: Readings in the Philosophy of Language* (New Jersey, Prentice Hall, 1964, p. 547).

Soviet citizen today who dissents is diagnosed and hospitalized as schizophrenic. Because he wants to change governmental policies, a Soviet dissenter is said to suffer from "reformist delusions." One can still be behavioral in orientation but assess, using overt external action as data, the behavior of internal structures and functions. It is computational behavior, operations of symbolic relations-structures, toward which we should direct our investigations. We must define the principles or rules of optimally well-functioning human computational systems.

Inquirer: You are cheerfully sidestepping the problem of generality and you are not too gracefully sidestepping the issue of a reference class. Human hardware of anatomy and physiology are generally similar throughout the world. Human software, mental processes, shows a bewildering diversity across cultures. A physical disorder is a physical disorder regardless of what the patient's culture defines as mental abnormality.

Psychiatric
Scientist: I am very surprised to hear you say this about physical disorder because it is a both narrow and ill-founded view. What is considered a physical disorder is equally dependent upon all sorts of cultural beliefs and practices. Since our views are rooted in Western-nation values and traditions about what is excellent, we tend to take our own biomedical norms as standards of defining physical disorder. Disease and disorder are theoretical constructs, abstractions from observations. There exists no universally valid view of what physical disease is or what its causes are.[24]

Inquirer: Surely, a broken leg or a cerebrovascular accident are recognized in all cultures as disorders.

Psychiatric
Scientist: Quite so. All cultures also recognize excessively violent or excessively grieving persons as disordered. These are the easy cases. The hard cases are those in

---

[24]See Fabrega, H.: Concepts of disease: logical features and social implications (*Perspectives in Biology and Medicine, 15*:583, 1972), as well as his, The function of medical-care systems: a logical analysis (*Perspectives in Biology and Medicine, 20*: 1976).

which cultural assumptions or theories about disease determine which properties are salient in characterizing disorders, what causes them, and what is to be done about them.

Inquirer: The Mind Scientist pointed out that many mental processes are artifactual in origin (i.e. they are man-shaped and man-guided). We are systems open to influence and perturbations not only by the physical environment, such as diet and climate, but also by the socio-symbolic environment that continuously penetrates and restructures our internal representations. We penetrate these environments and they penetrate us. We are members of both natural kinds and artifact kinds. If you are going to design an idealized mental system, it must contain elements based on rationality assumptions as to what is beneficial and what is harmful to human interests. Different groups of people have different values about what is beneficial and what is harmful. I don't see how you can set up universal norms for human mental functioning since a system always has a reference frame, something other than itself, that it accommodates to.

Psychiatric
Scientist: There exists no value-free criterion of functional normality for bodily systems either. In medicine, Murphy has been pursuing the "normal" all his life and still hasn't found it.[25] If we could set up criteria for *optimal*, we could forget the word *normal* altogether. We should limit ourselves to patterns, laws, and theories about particular reference classes just as evolutionary biology deems Mendel's laws to hold only for particular (not all) breeding groups. PARRY's pattern theory contains a law restricted to a kind, a circumscribed group of people suffering from paranoia. It doesn't bother me to think of defining mental disorder relative to a reference class without generalizing to the entire human population — past, present, and future. Because there are

---

[25]Murphy, E. A.: The normal, and the perils of the sylleptic argument (*Perspectives in Biology and Medicine, 75*:566, 1972).

	many shoe shapes and sizes does not imply there cannot be standards for a good shoe fit.

Inquirer:

I yield for the nonce. So you want to define mental disorder in terms of computational functions. I well understand that you can't observe computational functions. They are underlying mechanisms, not manifest properties. So how do you propose to study them in empirical mental systems?

Psychiatric
Scientist:

By making inferences about them using overt patterns of action as indicators of the underlying design. Most of what exists in the universe is not directly observable by us. But we can detect the effects of imperceptibles by detecting their signs. Humans are smart enough to have figured out there exist frequencies and wavelengths far beyond what we can see or hear. Infra-red radiation, gamma rays, and radio waves are good examples.

Overt actions of persons represent effects of processes we conceptualize at a representational level. We want to postulate the optimal functioning of these representational processes so that we can say the system is doing what it is supposed to do in approximate accordance with its ideal design. Psychologists, or someone, must provide psychiatry with the theoretical system-design of the proper working order of mental capacities at least for some reference classes in some population. What combination of variables optimizes mental activity in the ideal system? The theoretical system must be designed with an eye for constraints and limitations of mental activity

I assume the design problem will be investigated by exercising our available scientific methods of disciplined conjectures and imagination controllable and correctable by logic and empirical observations. The ideal design could even be taken as a standard for health-states that require no interventions. Empirically, no one would be totally mentally healthy because no actual individual meets all the idealized definitions of the optimal design. Then the question becomes one of deciding which departures from the ideal require remedial interventions. Empirical mental health would imply only that no penalities would ensue if interventions were *not* carried out.

Inquirer: Would you mean that proper or well-functioning is empirically "normal" in some statistical sense? Or do you mean the optimal would be the norm?

Psychiatric Scientist: One would like to approach near-optimality, the best approximation to an ideal achievable in a reference class.[26] If complete optimal health is taken as an ideal, no one is completely healthy physically or mentally because no one possesses full-optimality. Pragmatically speaking, order entails some degree of freedom from disorder. To borrow a concept from decision theory, we could talk about "satisficing," that is, what is good enough for an empirical system under its existing restrictions.[27] Satisficing means "towards optimal" to some satisfactory degree of approximation. For example, decision-makers never have complete information. They cannot foresee all consequences, and they are under pressure of time. So they make decisions that satisfice. They are not necessarily the best, but they are satisfactory and sufficient approximations given all the limitations.

In mental disorders, satisficing standards that determine whether remedial intervention is required are more appropriate than statistical norms. If statistical norms were used to determine abnormality, we would consider all left-handers "abnormal." Purely statistical norms for mental well-functioning are questionable because of the problem of the reference class.

---

[26]Living systems "normally" (i.e. usually) neither maximize nor minimize with full-blast capabilities. They approximate a near-optimality in a way that is best for the whole system, rather than utilizing the extreme operation of any subsystem, except in emergencies. The optimal is an extremum principle, a theoretical ideal to be approached and approximated but never actually achieved by actual empirical systems.

[27]This concept was first brought up by the Mind Scientist in Dialogue VI. See Simon, H.A.: *The Sciences of the Artificial* (Cambridge, MIT Press, 1969) for an extensive explication.

What is a normal serum cholesterol? Masai warriors have levels around 100, whereas American businessmen have levels of 200-300. If serum cholesterol were not known to be related to heart disease, these widely varying values would be considered abnormalities but not disease indicators. Pygmies and basketball centers may be abnormal, but they are not diseased.

Inquirer: What sort of evaluation would determine what is mentally satisficing and what is a mental disorder requiring intervention?

Psychiatric
Scientist: Since we currently lack a theoretical ideal design for the optimal function of mental systems, we must start over in the natural history phase of inquiry with a taxonomy that groups individuals, rather than grouping diseases or disorders. One would like to start from scratch, but then one would first have to invent the universe. In our domain, we first determine a reference class of individuals limited by age, sex, locations, occasions, and perhaps by additional variables. A satisficing representational or computational function, within members of this reference class, is one that makes a typical satisficing, near-optimal contribution to their individual adaptive and problem-solving strategies.

Notice that many, if not most, of the troubles we have in mental life concern other persons in the world whom we influence or perturb and by whom we are influenced or perturbed. Overall mental well-functioning represents the capacity and readiness of each computational function to perform on typical occasions with typical, but not necessarily maximal, efficiency in interactions with the physical and socio-symbolic environments. Satisficing functioning is relatively free of constriction or distortion by intrapersonal distress. A disorder represents an internal state that interferes with or reduces one or more saticficing computational functions below typical efficiency.[28] Treatment for such conditions would involve freeing an individual from a particular class of restrictions on near-optimal computational functions.

Inquirer:

Ow! My head hurts. What a trip! You have unloaded all sorts of new, vague and even question-begging concepts on me. What are all these notions about "typical," "adaptive," "problem-solving strategies," "readiness," "occasions," and "efficiency"?

Psychiatric
Scientist:

I am not about to unscramble all of them here. I can only refer you to some relevant literature.[29] But let me offer an example that illustrates these concepts in use. Let us assume mental representational functions enable us to acquire knowledge about the world. Representations are Peirce's "interpretants," construals of signs by an agent, the interpreter. Persons retain symbolic representations, models about their world of experience. Imagine these models as coarse conceptual sketches, good enough for us to get around with. A model is made up of symbolic components and has a structure relating the components to one another and to the environment. The relations-structure of the model does not mirror the structure of the world any more than the structure of the word *dog* mirrors the physical structure of a dog. Components of a model are codifications of elements in the world and in the individual himself allowing him to generate flexible, congruent and fitting accommodative behavior. A two-year-old child has a very limited, imperfect, gappy, ill-fitting and distorted model which, as he becomes an adult, becomes corrected, filled in, better fitted and

---

[28]Notice the Psychiatric Scientist, with uncharacteristic hesitancy, is offering definitions (and not very clear ones at that) rather than criteria. As we have heard, a definition gives the meaning of a concept. Criteria are tests which tell us whether a definition applies to a particular individual. What are the criteria for all these definitions?

[29]One place to start is in the writing of Boorse on the topic of health. See Boorse, C.: What a theory of mental health should be (*Journal for the Theory of Social Behavior, 6*:61, 1976), and Boorse, C.: Health as a theoretical concept (*Philosophy of Science, 44*:542, 1977). Also see Klein, D.F.: A proposed definition of mental illness. In Spitzer, R.L., and Klein, D.F. *Current Issues in Psychiatric Diagnosis*, p. 41.

greatly extended.

One essential computational function in an adequate (satisficing problem-solving) model involves making correct credibility assignments to belief propositions. For example, suppose I hold, with a high-credibility weight, the belief that Ronald Reagan is now (1983) president of the United States. To get by in the world I live in, I endorse this belief and make decisions (e.g. in voting) in accordance with it. If I held that James Carter were now president, said so to other people and behaved accordingly during election time, it would be justifiable to say something is wrong with me according to everyday rules of rightness. My key does not fit the relevant lock. I have made an incorrect, personally distorted credibility assignment. I now harbor a delusion, a false belief, a product of some inner personal distress with reasons of its own.

A clear example in psychiatry is paranoid states. Suppose a paranoid patient assigns a high credibility to the belief that the Mafia is trying to harm him. No one else endorses his belief. Fearing the Mafia, the patient behaves in ways that are atypical for his reference class. Trying to solve what, to him, are Mafia-related problems, he cannot solve the everyday problem of leaving his house at night. He barricades the doors and sits in his bedroom in the dark with a shotgun in his lap. Thus, we say he suffers a disorder because we infer there exists an interference with computational function of making correct credibility assignments. This results in an inability to perform typically (i.e. like other people in his reference class) on typical occasions (i.e. like going out at night). Does this make any sense to you?

Inquirer: Only some of it. I can buy the paranoid example because it is so obvious to everyone. But I am still bothered by the concept of mental well-functioning being related to membership in a reference class. Different reference classes have different normative values as to what is proper functioning. You will wind up with multiple ideal theoretical designs with varying constraints for different reference classes. Supposing all members of a reference class held a belief that members of another reference class took to be a delusion? Or suppose a fundamentalist group believed the world was only a few thousand years old and a member of this group accepted this belief. Is he mentally disordered because his belief is mistaken? Is his representational system not in proper working order?

Psychiatric
Scientist:

A very delicate question. How did he acquire this belief about the earth's age, and how does it bear on his computational capacities? The information is in error, but he may simply accept what he has been told and he does not challenge authority. He cares about the opinions and approval of members of his group. He does not complain that he is ill and no intervention is required. His erroneous belief simply reflects an inadequacy, which most of us have in some way or another. As a good fundamentalist, he is in no trouble. But if he were a professor of biology, he would have difficulties.

In contrast, a paranoid delusion represents an individual's *private* creation, an attempt to solve a problem of inner distress. A child fundamentalist may or may not change his belief when he grows up or when presented with contrary evidence. But a paranoid delusion is an affective *conviction*. It is not a corrigible belief that can be cognitively penetrated and shaken by evidence. Any counterevidence presented is transformed into positive evidence. The delusion is a solution to a painful problem having little to do with a congruence view of truth in which the outside patterns of facts correctly fit their internal representations. What for us, as observers, is a problem in the paranoid is, for him, *a solution* to a severely distressful problem, and he will not relinquish it until some other solution to his affective distress becomes available. We think being this way is not in his best interests as a well-functioning person, but he disagrees. His computational functions are hindered, reduced and distorted such that he can no longer adequately compute what are his best interests. His illness is stabilized and oscillates around a "norm" or equilibrium of its own. Paradoxically, it is a type of false health. Paranoids have false beliefs, but possession of false beliefs does not necessarily imply mental disorder.

I said the reference class was determined by age, sex, and "perhaps additional variables." Here you have a point. If one of the properties for membership in the reference class is a religious belief, then we are back into the morass of social praxis and conformity as arbiters of what is mental order and disorder. If members of a group believe in the devil, and one individual in that group does not, we should not say he is necessarily suffering from a disorder. He may have trouble accommodating himself to that group but may fit in with some other group. In a pluralistic society, there exists a variety of satisficing groups to be members of in which one does not suffer from interferences with computational functions.

Can we say that a large group of people share a mental disorder? I don't see why not. Consider the problem of the good Nazi. He fitted the norms of his limited socio-symbolic community but, according to us, committed crimes against humanity. Perhaps there are, or should be, universal values regarding the sanctity of all human life and respect for all human welfare. These questions are beyond my expertise. As I grow older, I find it easier to say "I don't know."

Inquirer: I would prefer the view that satisficing criteria are good enough for an individual. What is a satisficing approximation to the optimal for me may not be so for you. A treatment intervention that is good enough for me might make you worse off along some dimension.

Psychiatric
Scientist: But doesn't that mean we are members of different groups to which the intervention is applied? As the Academic Clinician indicated, therapy may result in a patient changing his group in order to increase his personal well-being and satisfying his best interests.

Inquirer: I think both you and the Biological Scientist, as professed realists, have a somewhat unrealistic and idealistic view of classes, groups, and kinds. Both of you realize that reference classes are abstractions, cognitive tools we use to solve problems in, and make sense of, the world. Both of you then think the classes of humans you construct refer to classes out there in the world existing as factual partitions or clumps in human nature independent of social praxis. You underestimate the force of the social normative in discriminating between mental order and disorder, rationality and irrationality. Classification schemes are man-made artifacts like hammers or bridges.

Psychiatric
Scientist: But the artifacts wouldn't be effective if they didn't somehow lock into and mesh with reality.

Inquirer: They don't have to fit reality in the sense of a point-to-point mapping or a one-to-one correspondence. Our models are partial matches. They have to connect to our world only coarsely or contact it globally to suit human purposes. It is human purposes behind a taxonomy which drives it to cluster things in one arrangement of kinds rather than another. The Biological Scientist points to species as an example of a concept which fits a real group in the world. But she admits the species concept is still very controversial. Biologists may eventually abandon it because of its limited application.[30] In psychiatry, you want groups or clusters which suit your purposes of management, treatment, prognosis, prevention and eventual understanding of the underlying mechanisms. Through interventions, you want to restore

---

[30]Some biologists believe in the reality of species, but the reality may be only apparent. See Levin, D. The nature of plant species. If you take six individuals and examine them along six morphological dimensions, you might cluster them into two groups based on these particular resemblances. If you used six chemical dimensions, you might wind up with three groups or four groups or one group. Which grouping is correct? It depends on your purposes. What is always overriding in a taxonomy are the purposes and interests of the taxonomist. It may be cognitively satisfying for one taxonomist to have two groups, whereas another taxonomist, preferring a greater refinement of granularity, chooses a larger number of groups. There are lumpers and splitters. Some biological taxonomists insist on sub-species and varieties below the species level, whereas others do not. This argument may seem a long way from classifying mental disorders, but it is not. Choices are involved.

disordered mental functions of individuals to within some satisfactory range. Using a dimensional scheme, you might find that patients can be clustered into five fairly homogeneous groups. Do any of the groups have clinical predictive utility? Would they respond successfully to the same management decisions? The subsequent clinical consequences of being in these groups might not be the same for the group members. You can have cognitive satisfaction in forming groups without necessarily attaining the long-run pragmatic satisfaction of the successful interventionist.

Psychiatric
Scientist: I can't accept that it is all that disconnected. We know there are syndromes in medicine that hold up even when the underlying mechanisms are discovered. Properties tend to hang together and drag one another along. Given properties P_1, P_2, and P_3 in an individual, there is a likelihood he will also possess P_4. And P_4 may be a response to an intervention or management decision similar to other individual people who have P_1, P_2, and P_3. Patterns, law-like relations, exist. Notice I said likelihood. These law-like relations represent tendencies and probabilities, not exceptionless timeless universals. How could medical syndromes be possible if the groups are arbitrary as you suggest?

Inquirer: I didn't say arbitrary, although Locke and Darwin implied that there was an element of conjecture to groups.[31] The real world is ordered, but the order can be looked at from a variety of perspectives and using a variety of conceptual levels. When you cut an apple

----

[31]Locke said: "Genera and species . . . depend on collections of ideas as men have made, and not on the real nature of things. . . . Our distinct species are nothing but distinct complex ideas, with distinct names annexed to them." See Locke, J.: *An Essay Concerning Human Understanding*, 1689, reprinted, J. W. Yolton (Ed.) (Dent, London, 1961). Although he entitled his book (*On the Origin of Species by Means of Natural Selection,*) Darwin stated therein: "I look at the term species as one arbitrarily given, for the sake of convenience, to a set of individuals closely resembling each other, and it does not essentially differ from the term variety which is given to less distinct and more fluctuating forms." And again, "We shall have to treat species as . . . merely artifical combinations made for convenience. This may not be a cheering prospect; but we shall at last be freed from the vain search for the undiscovered and undiscoverable essence of the term species." One of the great evolutionary biologists of our century, J. B. S. Haldane, stated: "The concept of a species is a concession to our linguistic habits and neurological mechanisms."

horizontally, a five-pointed star appears. Finer inspection depends on whether you are going to view the apple through a microscope (the star will disappear) or as a cellulose solution in a test tube (what star?). Which perspective and which level is a matter of our own choosing depending on our purposes. We can make the wrong choice, remember. Didn't psychiatrists once group certain patients under the heading "dementia praecox"? It turned out that many of these patients did not develop dementia, and many patients with the symptoms were not young. Hence, you had to form a different group of patients who did not deteriorate.

Psychiatric
Scientist: I think I see what you are getting at. At first, I thought you meant that by our clusterings, we were being entirely arbitrary in ordering the world. I can live with the idea that the way we cluster patients is partly a matter of our own choosing and partly a matter of some lawful properties they possess independent of us. I can agree our own contribution is essential and inseparable. When it comes to mental disorders, we have to find more properties that patients share, and we have to take the chance that some of the properties may be irrelevant to the patient's illness.

Inquirer: If you found five patients with persecutory delusions, four of whom were left-handed and red-headed, how would you decide on the relevance of handedness and hair color?

Psychiatric
Scientist: At last an easy question. In my own personal probability system, the *a priori* plausibility of handedness and hair color having any relevance for incorrect credibility assignments characteristic of persecutory beliefs would be low. The result you propose may be a sampling problem. But it should not be dismissed out of hand. If we had machine-readable records, we could study the data collected retrospectively looking for this pattern. Otherwise, we simply continue to collect cases of persecutory delusions to see if the initial

apparent syndrome holds up. If we begin to get eight out of eight or ten out of twelve, we begin to believe in a syndrome. If the association does not hold up as the sample size increases, we can say handedness and hair color are probably irrelevant to this disorder, or we can say we may have come across a rare syndrome and wait for additional examples to appear or be reported in the literature.

Inquirer: What concerns me about the view of mental illness you recommend is that it is still vague, the design question is unanswered, and you have no criteria for satisficing and non-satisficing mental functions. What are you going to do to improve this situation?

Psychiatric
Scientist: I didn't say *I* would do what should be done. But I do know someone who is trying to. He even has written several grant proposals about it. He is your man.

Inquirer: I must speak with this intrepid Grantsman.

THE GRANTSMAN

THE Grantsman is a research psychiatrist who spends much of his working time in the world of sponsored investigation, an endeavor that requires grant funds, sums of money for personnel salaries, space, equipment, subjects and miscellaneous facilities. To gain sponsorship, he must submit grant proposals to funding agencies, branches of the federal government, and private foundations. When a grant gets funded, the research work gets done. Otherwise it does not, and the Grantsman then fills his day with the writing and rewriting of proposals. He looks a bit forlorn and dispirited.

Inquirer: I hear from the Psychiatric Scientist that you have not only ideas but even a new method for improving the psychiatric classification system, and that you have submitted grant proposals regarding this method.

Grantsman: The Psychiatric Scientist is a friend and colleague of mine. We agree on many points but not on everything. If two people agree on everything, one of them is unnecessary. As we proceed, you will hear what some of the disagreements are.

Inquirer: So proceed.

Grantsman: My idea is not to try directly to improve the current DSM-III; it is to develop an *alternative* taxonomy.

Inquirer: People will say, "We still haven't got DSM-III straightened out, and here this wild man is running off trying to develop another taxonomy."

Grantsman: I quote the motto of a college at Aberdeen University: "They say what they say, let them say." But I will do more. I will give you my reasons.

When a field is progressing slowly, if at all, it may be that we are on the right path but not working hard enough at it. Or it may be we are on the wrong path, and we must back up in order to start in a

163

new direction. My feeling is we are not going to get any further with a long dynasty of DSM-II, III, IV, V, etc. based solely on juggling and rearranging signs and symptoms that have been known for centuries. This does not imply we should discard known signs and symptoms, but we must search for, and add, new properties to them. Another reason why the official scheme is so unreliable and unpromising as a guide to future research is that it groups properties intuited as relevant rather than grouping individuals based on systematic empirical inquiry. We need a method for grouping individuals on the basis of shared properties. It is hopeless to dream up sets of properties based on clinicians' intuitions and then try to fit individuals into them.[1] We need a systematic way to acquire new data, new manifestations, and new characteristics of disorder.

Inquirer: Do you have a new method of finding properties and grouping individuals?

Grantsman: I do. I think, first, we must start all over again with our initial problem situation. By thinking through our initial problem situation, we can re-analyze what it demands. How do we articulate, explore, and try to resolve our initial problem? One would like to start without presuppositions, but one never can. We are always aided and burdened by our predecessors' knowledge. Thinking is furthering the thinking of others. One builds on or transforms inherited views, received interpretations. Knowing something, we always want to know more. In the human and psychiatric sciences, we are enjoined not to use examples from physics because it looks too much like a case of borrowing prestige. But I will use one anyway, as did the Psychiatric Scientist.

Consider how Galileo approached the problem left by Aristotelian physics. Something was wrong with the traditional Aristotelian definition of force and Galileo realized a new concept was needed. The

---

[1]See Colby, K. M., and McGuire, M. T.: Signs and symptoms: zeroing in on a better classification of neuroses (*The Sciences*, 21:21, 1981).

problem was not the motion of projectiles, but any motion whatever. Galileo thought about the uniformly accelerated motion of falling bodies and tried to decide what the relevant factors were in such falls. He concluded that the velocity of the fall through space was proportional, not to the weight of the bodies or the distance, but to the elapsed time of fall. It took him about twenty-six years to make the correct decision. And he still didn't get it quite right because the value of the gravitational constant was not known at that time. In this way, force gained a new definition as that which produces, not velocity, but change of velocity or acceleration. The point of the story is that the initial stage of inquiry involves a reduction of the problematic situation to the relevant factual situation.[2] In psychiatry, we must re-analyze our initial problem situation, the situation which is generating our inquiry, to try to reduce it to relevant facts.

Inquirer: And what is that problematic situation?

Grantsman: It is the situation of someone being a patient and appealing to an expert for help. There is a job to be done by both participants. A patient feels he is ill in bodily or mental ways or both. Patients have troubles; they suffer; they have complaints; they feel ill; they want information and remedies. In the field of medicine, a patient's complaints are taken as indicators of disorder and an inquiry begins that is aimed at relieving the illness. The patient-expert complaint situation is where we should start again in psychiatry.

Inquirer: Aren't there mental disorders which do not produce complaints or suffering in the patient?

Grantsman: Even in medicine, a patient may not be aware of harboring a disorder. He may need help but not know that he needs help. A psychiatric patient may be troubled but not know it. To simplify things, let's just consider patients who are suffering and who

---

[2]The point and the example are from Northrop, F.S.C.: *The Logic of the Sciences and the Humanities* (New York, MacMillan, 1947). A comprehensive treatment can be found in Drake, S.: *Galileo at Work: His Scientific Biography* (Chicago, University of Chicago Press, 1978). A Galilean quip is that the Bible tells us how to go to heaven, but not how the heavens go.

consult experts. Persons have their own personal norms or standards of wellness. In psychiatry, a patient presents himself with complaints of troubles regarding his mental functioning that he has not always had. His own natural course of expected events has undergone a lapse. He is now experiencing some sort of symptom or incapacity, a personal discontinuity, a repeated or lasting deviation from his own norms. Something is wrong according to his personal norms of rightness. He seeks information about what is wrong, and he seeks to right it by consulting and communicating with those he takes to be informed experts in these matters. We need a taxonomy of mental unwellness before we get to a taxonomy of disorders.

Inquirer: You are relying heavily on the patient as an authority. What he believes to be wrong may not be wrong, or there may be nothing wrong with him at all.

Grantsman: The patient's view that he is ill has as good a right to be considered initially as yours or mine. We are starting with illness, a disorder in a host, and not with a disease, as was emphasized by the Old Psychiatrist.[3] We are stepping back to work in a theoretical vacuum at the initial pursuit stage of inquiry, the stage of classic pretheoretical empiricism. At this starting point, I am willing to adopt provisionally a philosophical principle of first-person epistemic authority. This mouthful means a person can usually be considered a good authority of his own inner subjective states of thoughts and feelings. Through self-awareness and L-consciousness, a person is a privileged observer of himself, having access to information no one else has. A person knows he is in pain, for example, in ways in which we cannot. Using ordinary language, he is in a priviledged position to give us an account of his mental sufferings and of his complaints. His accounts are informative communications intended for a receiver from whom benefit is expected. The Mind Scientist made clear the value of L-consciousness in

---

[3]In Dialogue II. The properties of the host are as important as the disorder in contributing to membership in an illness group.

communicating results of mental activity.[4]

Inquirer: The complainant is bringing himself to your attention. Since patients are self-selected, you don't really have a systematically drawn sample in the usual scientific sense.

Grantsman: Quite so. In a systematic investigation, a sample of a parent or universe population is selected according to a variety of sampling plans and studied. Further characteristics discovered about the sample are then generalized to the parent population. But if you don't know the characteristics of the parent population to begin with, you are in no position to sample it. Hence, we can *define* our starting collection or conglomeration of self-selected patients as the starting parent population, or reference population — a domain of individuals we are interested in (See Figs. 5 & 6).

Inquirer: Okay. As you discover further characteristics about the reference population and learn about its structure (i.e. the relationship between its individuals), you can begin to sample from *it* in the usual ways. You don't worry about bias or representativeness or sampling at the start because you cannot say what part of some larger population your collection is a sample of. Generalizations come later. The accounts you receive are first-hand descriptions by the person himself. Aren't they still open to all the traditional criticisms of introspective reports as being inaccurate and unreliable?

Grantsman: Yes, both I and the Mind Scientist admit this. Again, since we are in the starting phase, let's give the idea a little breathing room. Extreme behaviorists have claimed that introspective data are worthless. They overlooked the fact that one of the more "scientific" branches of psychology, namely, psychophysics, has long used such data in its experiments. The experimental subject indicates whether he sees or hears the stimulus by pressing a yes/no switch or saying "yes" or "no." He even

---

[4]Cf. Dialogue VI for the discussion with the Mind Scientist about L-consciousness — an awareness of some products of mental activity displayed linguistically in the auditory mode of inner speech and communicable to others in natural language.

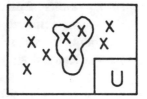

Figure 5. Picture a particular universe population as a rectangular space with *x*'s denoting individuals. Universe here does not mean the total population of the "universe" or world, but a small universe of discourse, a domain. The *x*'s included by the wavy line constitute a sample.

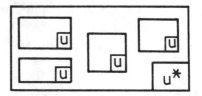

Figure 6. Like nested Chinese boxes, this small universe population can be combined with others to make up a larger universe (U*) and so on.

A sample of a universe or reference population is selected according to a sampling plan for which there are a variety of well-studied designs. Since he uses no systematic sampling plan at the start, the Grantsman stipulates his group to be a reference population.

describes what he sees (e.g. "yellow triangle," "red square"). This is introspective data reported by moving a finger or moving the mouth.[5]

Let me also remind you that first-person accounts have long been used in medicine to initiate inquiry into what might be wrong. Because he wants help, we assume patient is sincerely doing his best to provide authentic information. He may be overlooking some aspects of his mental states. But studies of psychiatric patients have shown that they are reliable, in the sense of being consistent over time, far more so than psychiatrists' judgments.[6] The pa-

---

[5]For a thorough treatment of the value of verbalized introspective data, see Ericsson, K. A., and Simon, H. A.: Verbal reports as data (*Psychological Review, 87*:215, 1980).

[6]See Ward, C. H., Beck, A. T., Mendelson, M., Mock, J. E., and Erbaugh, J. K.: The psychiatric nomenclature: reasons for diagnostic disagreement (*Archives of General Psychiatry, 16*:200, 1962). This study estimated that of the inconsistency in diagnosis, about 60 percent was due to DSM-II classification scheme, about 35 percent to the psychiatrist, and only 5 percent to the patient.

tient may be mistaken in some sense, but his own account may indicate what he is wrong about. Since a patient account is presented in ordinary language, it may represent an inadequate description of the descriptions in L-consciousness.[7] The patient may lack the vocabulary or skill of linguistic expression to accurately or sufficiently describe *to us* his lapse from wellness. Different patients may mean different things using the same words. Also, there are styles and degrees of linguistic eloquence. But a patient usually has a lot to say that is relevant to the purpose at hand. There is illness-relevant information in his communications and we should find the patterns expressed in his L-consciousness. Some of these description problems are alleviated when a psychiatric patient is allowed, on his own, to write out his first-person account of contents of L-consciousness.

Inquirer: Why does writing make a difference?

Grantsman: Face-to-face interviews present a well-known set of interferences in the collection of psychiatric patient data. Besides the interpersonal and status-differential problems between patient and expert, there are problems of interview structure. Over-structured interviews limit the patient to answering questions the expert has predetermined as being relevant. Under-structured interviews allow the patient to ramble all over topics whose relevance is questionable. We would like to have something in between which is both relevant and loosely structured and which minimizes the effects of our own physical-social-psychological presence on the patient's account. Hence, in addition to traditional interview data, I want to obtain a written account.

Inquirer: Won't a patient still ramble all over the place in his written account?

Grantsman: We impose a loose structure on a 2,000 + word account requesting four descriptions from him as follows:

(1) Describe your present life situation, your

---

[7]The descriptions appearing in L-consciousness, taken as *oratio recta*, may be transformed, paraphrased, or redescribed by *oratio obliqua* into the final linguistic output communicating ideas to others.

problems, and your thoughts and feelings about them.

(2)   Describe your thoughts and feelings about your work and/or school situation.

(3)   Describe your current most important personal relationship at this time.

(4)   Describe the most significant event in your life during the past year.

The job of writing out these descriptions gives a person a chance to organize his thoughts and to plan how he is to express them without being under the pace and pressure of a face-to-face interview. It is also interesting linguistically that written discourse is much easier for receivers to understand than oral discourse. Written discourse is more explicit and less ambiguous. Systematic studies have shown that oral discourse requires inferential propositions on the part of the listener at twice the rate of written discourse, and ambiguously placed propositions occur in oral discourse at *ten times* the rate of written discourse.[8]

Inquirer: How did you decide to request these four descriptions rather than some other set?

Grantsman: A question easier to ask than to answer. It seems one already has to know or assume something about what one is studying before one can study it. Galileo chose weight, distance, and time as factors in the free fall of bodies. Why didn't he choose color or shape as properties for study? There are plausibility constraints on what we take to be relevant versus meaningless properties. Our request set may turn out not to yield enough information for our taxonomic purpose, and we may have to change the topics of concern, but, at the initiation of inquiry, some a priori plausibilities are required. Psychiatric clinicians have long thought that information about interpersonal relations and work situations is relevant to mental disorder. I agree with them and with the Psychiatric Scientist who defines mental disorder

---

[8]See Deese, J.: Thought into speech (*American Scientist, 66*:314, 1978).

as a reduction or an interference with computational abilities to function typically on typical occasions at typical locations.[9]

Inquirer: Suppose you have collected these written accounts. What will you do with them? Will judges rate or score them in some way?

Grantsman: Not on your life. This has been a source of much of the past trouble in the classification scheme. If you turn human judges loose on these accounts, you will get a multitude of interpretations with few judges agreeing and a given judge giving a different interpretation on a different day. They have no uniform or consistent decision rules.[10] Our method involves having a computer algorithm analyze the accounts, looking for what we call conceptual patterns, key ideas, and themes that repeatedly express aspects of the patient's representational system. We want a standard, consistent way of analyzing accounts free of the unreliabilities, observer variations, and personal biases of human judges.

Inquirer: But didn't humans write the computer program? Doesn't it reflect their own biases?

Grantsman: Yes and no. This unsatisfying answer may become clearer as I describe how the algorithm works. The program looks at each word in each sentence of the account. A word designates a concept or, more precisely, a web or net of concepts that have meaning. Meaning consists of sense (intensional definition) and reference (the extensional set of things that satisfy the definition). The whole structure of the word-conceptual net is the signification of the word-symbol. Since meaning is a property of the conceptual net, words are vehicles having meaning indirectly or vicariously.[11]

---

[9]See Dialogue VIII for the discussion of mental disorder in terms of an interference with optimal computational functions.

[10]See Stoller, R. J., and Geertsma, R. H.: The consistency of psychiatrists' clinical judgment (*Journal of Nervous and Mental Disease, 137*:58, 1963). This instructive study reveals that it is not just diagnoses that the clinicians disagree about. They are highly inconsistent over a wide range of judgments involved in everyday clinical decision-making.

[11]The meaning of "meaning" is still elusive. For ten different definitions, see Cherry, C.: *On*
→

The algorithm tries to construct conceptual patterns from the words of the sentence, converting words and phrases into concepts and then connecting the concepts into a pattern. The conceptual patterns are combinations of concepts (e.g. they usually, but not invariably, consist of a subject and one or more predicates). Many are propositional attitudes consisting of a concern ("I fear") and a topic of concern ("that I will fail"). The conceptual patterns represent the senses and references of concepts designated by word-symbols.[12]

Inquirer: But you, the researchers, decided on what concept-structure a word designates and what the sentences signify in terms of combinations of concepts. Others might not agree and claim a given sentence signifies something else. The algorithm reflects biases about word and sentence meaning.

Grantsman: A research group does not decide arbitrarily what a word means. It leans on prior knowledge from those generations of workers who have spent hundreds of years in constructing English dictionaries and thesauri. The algorithm I am describing is solidly based on this scholarly knowledge of common standard usage of English. If you look at a thesaurus, say Roget's, you will find that a word has several synonyms and antonyms grouped under concepts.[13] A synonym is a

---

Human Communication (New York, John Wiley, 1957). Besides the signification of a symbol (semantic meaning), there is its significance (pragmatic meaning) involving the effect the sender of a message intends to produce in its receiver. The effect produced in the receiver may or may not correspond to the sender's intention. For more on these distinctions, see Morris, C. *Significance and Significance*, as well as Ackoff, R. L., and Emery, F. E.: *On Purposeful Systems* (Chicago, Aldin-Atherton, 1972). See also Searle, J.R.: *Speech Acts: An Essay in the Philosophy of Language* (Cambridge, Cambridge University Press, 1969).

[12]For some details as to how this parser works, see Parkison, R. C., Colby, K. M., and Faught, W. S.: Conversational language comprehension using integrated pattern-matching and parsing (*Artificial Intelligence*, 9:111, 1977), as well as Colby, K. M., Modeling a paranoid mind, p. 519. A complete description can be found in Parkison's dissertation, Parkison, R. C.: *An Effective Computational Approach to the Comprehension of Purposeful English Dialogue* (Department of Computer Science, Stanford University, 1980).

[13]For some deep insights into Roget, see Masterman, M.: Braithwaite and Kuhn: analogy clusters within and without hypothetico-deductive systems in science. In Mellor, D. H. (Ed.): *Science, Belief, and Behaviour* (Cambridge, Cambridge University Press, 1980). Most users of Roget's thesaurus do not even notice the design principles underlying its structural organization. For some opaque reason, they are not described explicitly in the volume itself.

word of similar meaning. Similarity means same but with a difference, otherwise there would be no need for two words. An antonym is a word of contrasting meaning, not necessarily directly opposite. No word is exactly synonymous or antonymic to another word.

In constructing our algorithm, we used the concepts and similarity-contrast words found in several standard thesauri and dictionaries available to us. We assume patients share the meanings of common usages. (Otherwise we would not understand them at all.) It was not our personal bias which decided that, for example, "fear" and "anxiety" are closely related words in a semantic space designating a similar conceptual structure. We found this relation in every work we consulted. Hence, we incorporated in the algorithm this high degree of agreement achieved by scholars of English. If someone constructs another algorithm that does not semantically relate "fear" to "anxiety," he would fly in the face of a widespread consensus, and he would have to justify his position on his own grounds.

Inquirer: But how about words over which the English scholars disagree? How do you decide on their meaning?

Grantsman: Touché. Disagreements occur, but they are not severe to the point of being antonymic. The greatest problem we have with thesauri is simply omission of words and phrases as exemplified in current popular usages or idioms which have not yet reached the thesauri. For example, "pork out" does not appear in published thesauri yet. (It means to gorge oneself, to make a pig of oneself.) In these cases, we do just what former scholars have done. I and my associates negotiate agreements and decide on what conceptual structure a word or phrase designates in its context. A word-symbol is always an incomplete vehicle for the representation of its represented conceptual net which is a much more complex structure of relations.

Our decisions reflect our personal judgments as native and skilled users of language in psychiatric contexts. Another group of workers might well propose a different signification for a word. But how different would it be and how much difference would the difference make in the overall run ? We would have to compare our algorithm with theirs on the same patient accounts. The important point is that the algorithm must be consistent and uniform, serving as a standard. As in physics, initially it may be an arbitrary choice as to what is left and what is right, and what is North and what is South, but once made, the decision stays the same for everybody during a time interval. It is a relative, not absolute, invariant. Our algorithm is applied to each patient account in exactly the same way and gives the same results when applied to a given account repeatedly.

Inquirer: How does your method differ from simple key-word searching?

Grantsman: A key-word search looks for certain words at the surface-level of linguistic expressions and counts them as instances of categories. Content analysis assigns words to a special dictionary of categories that can be viewed as concepts. The program then outputs the frequency of words in each of the categories.[14] The key-word searches we know about do not combine the concepts into higher level similarity-contrast patterns as our algorithm does. Key-word searches and content analysis deal mainly with single category terms. We are interested in the properties of the patient's messages, combinations of linguistic symbols constituting a sign-complex of constituents. The significance of a message lies not just in a sum of properties of individual constituent symbols but in the interactions of the symbols in a sign-complex, a message the algorithm decodes into a combinatorial, conceptual pattern. Since a conceptual pattern involves a complex of several constituent concepts, it provides richer semantic structures for analysis than does a simple key-word counting procedure.

---

[14]See Stone, et. al., *The General Inquirer*. For a recent study using this method, see Oxman, T. E., Rosenberg, S. D., and Tucker, G. J.: The language of paranoia (*American Journal of Psychiatry*, *139*:275, 1982). This study also offers evidential support for the shame-induced distress theory of paranoia embodied in the model PARRY discussed by the Mind Scientist in Dialogue VI.

Inquirer: Could you give me some examples of phrases or sentences which are considered instances of a conceptual pattern?

Grantsman: Each of the following actual surface expressions from the same patient account are taken to be similar in signification by the algorithm because they involve synonymic references to "fear": "My fear is that I won't have it even then"; "I'm not sure what the fears are about"; "The gnawing anxiety"; "Panic and insecurity"; "The fear constant"; and "My biggest fears have always been of being like her." They are all converted into the conceptual pattern "I fear."

Inquirer: Suppose you now have a lot of these conceptual patterns from an account. What do you then do with them?

Grantsman: The algorithm then clusters the conceptual patterns together on the basis of similarity-contrast relations between them. To simplify the terminology, I will label the clusters "key ideas" (KI). We are currently using about sixty key ideas. These more abstract clusters of key ideas are groups of recurrent conceptual patterns. A key idea is a *cluster* of conceptual patterns having similar or contrasting significations.

Inquirer: For example?

Grantsman: If you examine the expressions instancing the conceptual pattern that I have just quoted, you will see they all relate to "fear" but not to any contrast such as "security." A key idea is composed of all the conceptual patterns which relate to a dimension (labeled for our convenience only, "fear-security") through similarity and contrast relations which can be viewed as two ends of the dimension. For example, the following expressions, from the same patient account, would be clustered with those above to form key idea 22, an arbitrary label for the entire structure: "Yet everytime I could opt for security"; "Sitting next to a friend for comfort"; "Little or no worry about school"; "No worry about what I will do then." Each key idea is assigned a percentage rating according to the frequency of its appearance in the account compared to other key ideas. Imagine each key idea (KI) as a bar in a bar graph (see Fig. 7). One can then construct a profile, a pattern of recurrent themes, key ideas, that characterizes each person. Notice it is not the absolute frequency of a key idea which is important but the *ratio* of a key idea to all other key ideas. The final step is to cluster similar profiles into groups which would then yield groups of individuals sharing the property of similar KI profiles. This clustering is performed by readily available standard clustering algorithms.[15] Notice also we are grouping individuals according to their shared profiles. We do not first set up profiles and try to fit individuals to them, and we do not say the individuals have the same "disease." We are dealing with resemblance classes based on shared properties, not with diagnostic categories.

Inquirer: Your mention of the word *theme* reminds me of the Thematic Apperception Test, long used by psychologists. How does your procedure differ?

Grantsman: The Thematic Apperception Test consists of a selected set of pictures shown to subjects who compose and orally report stories about them. The narratives are scored by human judges according to theoretically predetermined characteristics or themes, such as references to competition and achievement. The test was not used to construct a taxonomy of mental disorders but to characterize personality. In our method, the thematic key ideas derive from the conceptual patterns of written accounts generated by the subjects themselves in response to information requests. The scoring is done by an algorithm, which forms profiles, and the profiles are clustered by another algorithm into resemblance groups, individuals sharing similar profiles.

---

[15]A good review of useful clustering algorithms can be found in Mezzich, J. E., and Solomon, H.: *Taxonomy and Behavioral Science* (New York, Academic Press, 1980). See also Everitt, B.S.: *Cluster Analysis* (London, Heineman Educational Books, 1974) as well as Skinner, H.A.: Dimensions and clusters: a hybrid approach to classification, (*Applied Psychological Measurement, 3*:327, 1979).

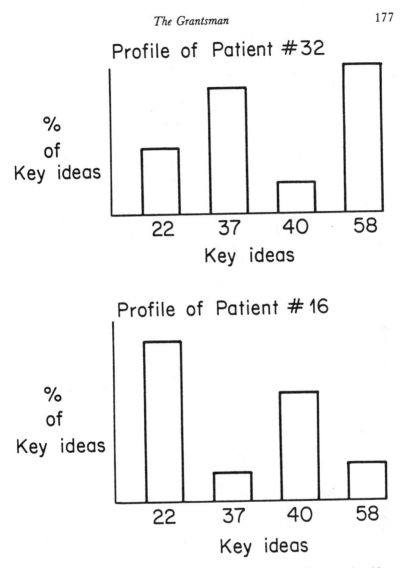

Figure 7. These two patients exhibit quite different profiles for the same key ideas.

Inquirer: The individual differences between people might be so great that groups could not be formed based on these patterned profiles.

Grantsman: Everyone shares some properties with someone else; there are *kinds* of people and *kinds* of dysfunctioning people. One can always form groups of some sort. The crucial question is whether the groups have purposive and predictive value. Are they natural or rele-

vant kinds as described by the Biological Scientist?[16]
A group might be useful for one purpose but not for
another. We are interested in the clinical *consequences*
of membership in the groups. Clinical, natural kinds
are formed for future-oriented management decisions and purposes. We and the patients want to
know what is likely to happen to them and what *ought
to be done* about it. Eventually, we would like to know
something about mechanisms that generate particular key ideas. A classification system should
generate further hypotheses about what causally produced and what now maintains the taxonomic ordering under a causal propogation.[17] Knowledge of the
generating mechanisms can eventually lead to a revision of the initial taxonomy enabling it to be based on
theoretical rather than empirical grounds. It becomes
redescribed in terms of a more theoretical vocabulary.

Inquirer: Suppose you can cluster patients with similar
profiles into groups. The groups may be reliable in
the agreement sense, but how will you know the
groups have any consequent clinical utility?

Grantsman: Research breeds research. One might first look at
groups now known to have a satisfactory degree of
reliability to see whether they correlate with any of
the groups formed on the basis of theme profiles.
The category "being paranoid," in the sense of possessing persecutory delusions, is very reliable as you have
heard.[18] Would patients characterized clinically as
paranoid belong to a group we might label (using
neutral terms) *Group IV* in our clustering system?

Inquirer: Why not try to correlate your groups with the DSM-
II or DSM-III categories?

Grantsman: It wouldn't surprise me if some correlations showed
up. But if they didn't, it wouldn't mean much
because the majority of these categories are known
to be unreliable. Another way of demonstrating ap-

---

[16]Natural kinds are those natural for us, as the Metaphysician emphasized.
[17]For this heuristic function of classification systems in furthering investigation, see Sokal, R.:
Classification: purposes, principles, progress, prospects (*Science, 185*:1115, 1974).
[18]See note 23 in Dialogue VI.

plicative utility would be to close the loop by showing that specific groups responded similarly to similar management decisions, such as a specific treatment (see Fig. 8). Treatment response would increase our confidence that we have relevant kinds. This way of closing a feedback coupling must await an initial grouping. First, we want to find out whether we can characterize patients according to the profiles of their key ideas, products of computational functions carried out in a representational system. Notice also we discover which key ideas a patient does *not* have in comparison to others. The holes in Swiss cheese are important defining properties.

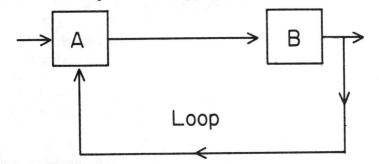

Figure 8. This example illustrates the concept of closing the loop to describe repeated cycles of processes in which there is feedback from one process occurring at time *t* to another earlier process at time *t-1*.

The output from process B is fed back as input to process A whose output feeds forward to process B. In an applicative cycle, in which an intervention is applied to members of a group, the results of the intervention "reciprocates" information regarding a new property for a reappraisal of the composition of the group. The cycle can be iterated or repeated indefinitely using various interventions or other management decisions.

Inquirer: You said now that you agree with the Psychiatric Scientist who suggested we should view mental disorders in terms of restrictions, limitations or interferences with optimal-approaching satisficing computational functions.

Grantsman: I do. What we are here calling a *key idea* represents a cluster of conceptual patterns that have been repeatedly activated in the account. They can be viewed as salient or regnant ideas that result from recurrent internal computational processes in the patient and serve as indicators of the patient's model-representation of his world of experience. It is not new to say patients with mental disorders have unusual ideas or peculiar concerns that preoccupy them. What is new here is that we have a systematic and consistent method of characterizing semantically and quantifying specifically what these ideas are, using a computer algorithm. We are inserting an instrument between the patient and the clinician to reduce the effects of his personal subjectivity on the factual objects of patients' descriptions. The method has greater "semi-objectivity." It has also internal validity (i.e. when it is repeated on the same data, it gives consistent and coherent results).[19]

Inquirer: I realize that nothing will ever get done if all possible objections must first be overcomes so this is a minor cavil at this point. Let's concede you can abstract a profile from the raw narrative data of a patient account. However, if you repeated the procedure six weeks or six months later, you might obtain an entirely different profile or pattern of key ideas.

Grantsman: That is a possibility which deserves study. A lot can happen in six weeks or six months to change a person's concerns. Patient-states are stochastic and may fluctuate over time. To date, we have only one example studied a year later. It was a case of paranoia in which the second profile, constructed one year after the first, was the same except for one dimension. In more volatile and less chronic conditions, changes are to be expected. But which key ideas change and which do not, and by how much? Your question can only be answered by empirical investigation and new data.

Inquirer: Your method might be picking up unusual or high-frequency key ideas that characterize a kind of person but may have nothing to do with a mental

---

[19]The Grantsman's method reflects a general strategy in the sciences of applying a mathematical formalism to an empirical domain. In real life, we have some troubles we do not know how to handle very well. We also have puzzles, mathematical formalisms, which have clear and sometimes elegant solutions. Science and technology specifically formulate a problem by finding an appropriate puzzle form to impose on a trouble. Solving the problem may allow us to handle the trouble better.

disorder. Properties that co-exist in an individual may not be relevant to one another. Ideas that just have to do with being a person may show up.

Grantsman: To answer this question, we must be able to compare accounts from patients with accounts from non-patient controls. We then subtract out the key ideas patients and controls have in common since these are ideas involved in just being a person. Irrelevant and incidental properties can always show up. Initially, we want to take any property seriously as a potential characteristic for a clinically relevant kind. Recall our working concept of unwellness as a disorder possessed by a host. Certain kinds of hosts may be vulnerable to certain kinds of disorders. The properties of the host are important for prognosis as well as treatment. You don't treat an eighteen-year-old high school student who believes he is Jesus Christ the same way you treat a sixty-year-old bank president who believes he is Jesus Christ. Over time, incidental properties will become empirically identified by their irrelevance for group membership.

In a small pilot study with 31 experimental subjects and 15 controls, we noticed that none of the control profiles showed a frequency of key ideas greater than 1-2 percent whereas in all complainant accounts of the experimentals, there were elevated peaks on several key ideas, some as high as 15 percent. Also, we have been able to cluster three distinct subgroups in the experimental group. The samples are still too small. But at least it suggests that if your patient is showing a high concern over his job situation, then it may be a manifestation of some sort of non-well-functioning in that area.

Inquirer: But why wouldn't a clinician simply pick this up in his interviews with the patient?

Grantsman: He might do so if the patient emphasizes it and if the clinician attends to it. As a human observer, the clinician has blind spots, deaf spots, and limited information-processing capacities. As you have heard, humans are not good recognizers and counters of multiple pieces of information. They can handle only about four, plus or minus two, "chunks" of information at a time.[20] A clinician might pick up a few key ideas, but not all of them, and patients can have many of them. He may consider a key idea to be salient when it is not of significant frequency. He has no sound way of quantifying key ideas. Because of observer variation, he might select different ideas as outstanding on different occasions of evaluating the same account. Also, he might not notice what ideas are *not* present. Humans are not good at utilizing negative information.[21]

Inquirer: I can see further uses for this method. High-percentage key ideas may indicate areas of concern toward which therapy might be directed in any patient. Another use of such a profile might be to follow treatment responses in terms of change in the individual's profile over time. What I mainly like about your method is that it potentially provides a breakthrough for dealing with the typical mountains of indigestible narrative data psychiatric patients present us. This problem of raw data reduction and finding semantic regularities has always plagued psychiatric research. We can handle demographic data and test scores easily, but if that is all we have, we have lost a great deal of information about the patient. Systematically analyzing what the patient describes about his thoughts and feelings should provide a rich source of manageable patient information. The inquiry procedure you have outlined seems a reasonable try to me. Why don't you go ahead with a full-scale research project?

Grantsman: Alas, and even alack! No funding. A project like this requires a skilled programmer and statistician, a computer and someone like myself in a clinical setting. All of these elements require money to exist. Like other current infantrymen of science, I have applied for grants and been rejected dozens of times.

---

[20]See Simon, H.: How big is a chunk?
[21]See Wason, P.C. and Johnson-Laird, P.N.: *Psychology of Reasoning.*

When does one abandon an idea? The research life is a mixture of enjoyment and despair, of swamps and meadows. The joy comes from working on your ideas; the despair comes when no one will provide the support necessary to work on your ideas. Repeated proposal rejection has corrosive effects on the morale of a research team and eventually dissolves it. But that is another story we can take up in the free-for-all.

Inquirer: What free-for-all?

Grantsman: In the final go-around, everybody will have his final say, including myself. So let's join the others and enter the fray.

Dialogue X

EVERYBODY TALKS

Inquirer:

Since I began all this, perhaps I should try to close down the argument with some sort of resounding conclusion.

Old
Psychiatrist:

Before you get to that improbable point, I would like to bring up a question or two. A "key idea" of our own dialogues seems to be that we need new data and new properties of disorder in psychiatry if we are to progress in solving the problems of the field. We need further facts about the initial problem situation. Then the Metaphysician suggested, however, that we do not deal with facts but with interpretations. This bothers me because for years in psychiatry, we have been saddled with divergent interpretations as to "what the patient meant" by something he said or did. I have been marched through all the usual pieties of the field, and I realize our experience has been that we get even fewer agreements about interpretations than we do about diagnoses.[1] How will we progress if our facts consist merely of interpretations, of opinions, about which we cannot agree?

Metaphysician:

It seems we have been using the term *interpretation* in two senses here: (1) the interpretation of signs resulting in their acquiring significance; and (2) interpretations by observers of other people's behavior. Interpretations in this second sense makes all the human sciences, as well as psychiatry, difficult. What I have been calling interpretations here are those in the first sense, and

---

[1] See Stoller and Geertsma, Consistency of psychiatrists' clinical judgement (p. 138). Why this study had such little impact on the field is a mystery only to those who do not understand how professional allegiances work.

they are not quite what you clinicians call an interpretation. If we observe a person's overt behavior and characterize this observation under some description, we have what is conventionally called a *fact*. Observer facts or data are phenomena read and described in a certain way.

Young
Psychiatrist: But more facts mean more interpretations. Aren't we in a circle here?

Mind
Scientist: No more so than any other science. Take physics again. Suppose you enter a physicist's study and see him staring at some photographs. How would you characterize what he is doing? At a common-sense level, you might say he is looking at photographs. If you ask the physicist what he is doing, he might say he is looking at an electron. If you ask where is the electron, he might say he is not really looking at an electron but at a photograph of its ionized vapor path in a bubble chamber. If you ask what the photograph has to do with an electron, he will reply that the structure of the vapor path in the photographs is isomorphic with the path of the electron that occurred in the chamber. If you ask what a vapor path is, he will probably give up this level of describing what he is doing because he realizes you do not have the stock of background knowledge needed to understand what he is talking about.

This stock of knowledge consists of hundreds of such characterizations and explanations built up over hundreds of years, one leading to another and the whole system converging into a dense, coherent conceptual network passed on by one generation of physicists to the next.[2] In a given field, in one context, a theory term can be taken

---

[2]This is what Kuhn means by a "disciplinary matrix" made up of symbolic generalizations, shared values, models, and exemplars of a field's scientific activity. See Kuhn, *Structure of Scientific Revolutions* (p. 182).

as an empirical term and vice versa. An *electron* can be both a theory term, an abstract entity, and an observation term, a fact packed with perceptual judgments. There are grades of theoreticity to terms.

Metaphysician: The dense, coherent conceptual network you refer to bears some resemblance to a metaphysical system, in that it provides a matrix within which facts can be assigned meaning. Most metaphysical systems are of greater scope and are specified in less detail than the conceptual network of most disciplines; on the other hand, the conceptual network of many disciplines seems to rest upon the assumptions of several different, often conflicting metaphysical systems. As I suggested earlier, realism and pragmatism appear to be adequate metaphysical systems for the brand of science you advocate for psychiatric research. But it could be different. Several metaphysical systems allow for the attainment of knowledge about the world by systematic inquiry. I suspect some of the participants in this dialogue hold to other views than realism and pragmatism.

Academic
Clinician: I guess I would be an example. In my clinical research I have tried to respect and hold to the requirements of rigorous "scientific method," basing my convictions on textbook canons of evidence generally accepted in the scientific community. But what I believe is real is only "experience" taken in the sense of "raw human awareness." My categories remain experiential at all times. This allows me to avoid a lot of ontological and epistemological conundrums and seems to allow a certain flexibility and openness in my belief structure. In short, I am willing to "take it as it comes."

Psychiatric
Scientist: What you call "real" raw awareness, I would call mere phenomenological appearance subject to indenumerable errors. The real lies beyond

manifest conscious experience; the real consists of independent imperceptible patterns with the power to generate manifest observable patterns.

Mind
Scientist:

The term *objective* nowadays does not mean quite what it meant to early twentieth century positivists. I previously defined *objective* as an intersubjective agreement fixed by the relevant expert forum over a time interval with respect to some system regardless of an observer's own personal preferences or views. Perhaps *semi-objective* would be a more acceptable term to you, implying the objective is at least half us. Intersubjective semi-objectivity is not *im*personal, but *multi*personal.

Academic
Clinician:

To me, a "real objective world" is a way of expressing a complicated quality of experience, something like: things get in my way . . . I can't budge some things . . . the world *objects*, as it were.[3] As I study my experience I learn more and more about tendencies in it, and I am led eventually to posit the existence of a "real world" as opposed to, say, "the world of fantasy," where I seem to be able to move around quite easily. For

---

[3]Peirce commented on this capacity of objects to object to us: "The properties of the world resist our will to make them other than they are so we must learn how they are." Peirce, *Collected Papers*. But "how they are" is highly dependent on what they are construed or characterized by us in a context. "A rose is a rose is a rose" (G. Stein). A gold ring is a gold ring. (Already these are characterizations.) Is a gold ring a piece of jewelry, a work of art, an article of commerce, an exhibit in a law suit, a token of marriage? Different significances are bestowed on the gold ring, meanings that cannot be comprehended by sensation alone. Sensors receive information; the information becomes converted, by higher-order processes, into perceptual judgments and beliefs.

The example is clear in the case of artifacts such as jewelry, ornaments, utensils, machines, tools, languages and paintings. But recall the Mind Scientist's remark asserting that many human representations — desires, beliefs, ideas, actions, attitudes, and emotions — are artifact kinds and thus mental tools. Kant used the term *representation* to designate a play. We can re-present to ourselves the deliverances of our own experiences. We (our systems) are the authors of our own representations, as well as being characters in them and an audience and critics of them. Artifacts can be works of art as well as machines. Our representations, derived from our own choices among alternative interpretations of signs, are in a sense autobiographical works of art.

me, "things," the "real world," "mind," "time," all of the referents of all of these symbols are simply qualities that I categorize verbally according to degrees of similarity. Things that I call "mental" *feel* different, and consistently different, from things that I call "physical," for example. But no qualities are ever identical for me, so I am not committed to believe in any static world structure. For all I know, it changes constantly. Practically speaking, though, I seem to be able to apply certain procedures in these times when I feel "stuck" so that I get "unstuck" and my experience flows again. You may call these procedures "solutions" to "problems" based on "laws" I have learned about the "real, objective world" by scientific method, if you choose, but I prefer not to. I have no particular need to deny any regularity that appears in my experience, and I'm even open to the possibility that there are "things out there" that can be "classified." I just don't assume that it *must* be so.

Inquirer:
Academic
Clinician:

Isn't that solipsism?

Hardly. I find it extremely useful to acknowledge the apparent existence of other people and find it equally expedient to consult them in certain matters. In fact, when it comes to "getting unstuck" in certain circumstances (those that involve the "objective world"), I find their opinions extremely valuable.

Metaphysician:

Several types of lawfulness or regularities can be imagined. For example, what if the universe is a continuously evolving structure, like the embryo of an organism, developing from embryonic to adult forms, so that new structures and relationships emerge through time. If you introduce time into the equations of physics, causality goes out the window because the concept of cause requires a non-evolving system in which the same state always gives rise to another same state and a *ceteris paribus* clause (all other things being equal) in addition. Evolution may itself evolve. What if it were possible to grasp the underlying direction of an evolving structure? This may lead to useful knowledge but would imply no sort of classification of kinds. Or what if the universe were a big machine, with each individual object being in the relation of part-to-whole rather than in a simple relation of class membership? Instead of being composed of tiny particles in motion, maybe the universe consists of tiny computers processing information. Maybe what we call *objects* are simply sets of instructions to carry out these activities that result in the objects' manifest properties. We say we model the world, but the world itself may be a model.[4] Suppose the universe is a big animal, with its own will and we are just cells and parts of cells in this animal. The Indians did quite well with a metaphysical system that interpreted the world as an animal.

Biological
Scientist: You say "well," but by what criteria? They weren't trying to solve difficult scientific or technical problems of the magnitude we are.

Metaphysician: Right! And you, as a scientist anyway, are not trying to achieve a sense of harmony with your environment. The historical context is different. You have new methods available and a different set of problems to solve, so your metaphysics is correspondingly different. No better, or more true, or less chaotic. Just different.

Mind
Scientist: I'm not sure I agree that we are *not* trying to

---

[4]The view that the world itself may be a representation (to whom? to what?) comes close to Berkeley's view of reality (that which exists), according to which the material world did not exist. Berkeley maintained that reality consisted only of our own conscious perceptions, of ideas that existed ultimately in God's mind. By "ideas," however, he meant only mental imagery. See Berkeley, G.: *Three Dialogues Between Hylas and Philonous in Opposition to Skeptics and Atheists*, 1725 (London, Everyman's Library, 1946).

achieve a harmony with our environment. There is more to harmony than control and influence. We want to understand the world and life not just for technological reasons but also to enjoy it, enhance it and appreciate it aesthetically as much as one would a Gothic cathedral. I think this is what scientists mean when they talk about the cognitive or intellectual satisfaction of their work, apart from pragmatic satisfaction. The practice of science itself is an art, and some of its products we view in simple awe as "beautiful." You make it sound like its all a cut-and-dried busyness *about* something without appreciating and enjoying the something as well.

Metaphysician: I yield to the emendation, which is little recognized publicly, but quite apropos. Perhaps because I have been talking to psychiatrists who are practitioners rather than scientists, I have overemphasized technological aspects. My main point was to stress the variety of legitimate metaphysical views that are conjectures as much as scientific theories are.

Psychiatric
Scientist: You mean any metaphysical belief is as *valid* or as *rational* as any other?

Metaphysician: Not at all. Systems and world versions vary in many ways.[5] Some account for more of man's experience than others. Some are more precise in their specification of experience. Some are more aesthetically pleasing than others. Some are "conservative," and some "liberal," etc.

Psychiatric
Scientist: Politics and aesthetics?

Metaphysician: Sorry. But doesn't a crystalline world of unchanging "forms" and "universals," of "substance" and "essence," or one of "everlasting fire" have more

---

[5]See Goodman, N.: *Ways of Worldmaking* (Cambridge, Hackett, 1978). Goodman is a nominalist, who denies the existence of universals and classes, but at times he wavers toward realism in speaking of "fair" samples of a pattern that may apply to a whole of further samples. Also see Stephen C. Pepper's classic *World Hypotheses* (Berkeley, University of California Press, 1970).

appeal than one of "malevolent will"? This difference in aesthetic appeal may account, in part, for the greater historical impact of Aristotle's thought, and Heraclitus', than Schopenhauer's. And, yes, there are political differences in metaphysical systems. Conservatives have political beliefs based on resistance to change ("paradise is now"), whereas liberals have always looked to change as a key to the future, when the "lot of man" will be better. Some metaphysics, for example, have no category for true novelty. They assume that all phenomena are bound by universal laws that are immutable for all time. The Academic Clinician here, however, can grant the reality of "inexplicable" occurrences. The implications should be clear.

Biological
Scientist:

To be frank with all of you at this point, other scientists do not expect much to happen in the way of progress in the human behavioral sciences or even in psychiatry. Both fields lack an agreed-on taxonomy of non-vague categories, they can't agree on what they are talking about, and their methods of arriving at agreement have not been very successful. It is a scientific research program based on, and proceeding from, a first step of a reasonably reliable taxonomy that becomes productive of "useful truths," if you'll pardon the expression.

Psychiatric
Scientist:

Careful, you're preempting a justification from my system, namely, usefulness. The proper justification for "truths" generated by your brand of science are degrees of fit between the meaning of propositions and the world about which they are asserted. To me truths are true only as long as they are useful cognitively or pragmatically. They are empirically adequate, as $truth_2$, not necessarily $truth_1$ reality, and no correspondence to $truth_1$ is required or assumed.

Mind
Scientist: It has been claimed that the behavioral sciences
will never provide reliable scientific knowledge.
For example, Ziman, a physicist, maintains that
scientific statements have two properties, consensibility and consensuality.[6] By the first property,
consensibility, he means that the statements are
intelligible and have a clear meaning for
equivalent observers. Scientific discourse presupposes conditions for unambiguous communication of information. If a statement is consensible
and affirmable, it is a potential candidate for consensus regarding its truth. He doubts if the
human sciences can ever generate statements
with these properties. There are too many
disagreements about what human behavior
statements mean, let alone whether they are true.

Metaphysician: I am more optimistic. The human sciences need
more time, more bright people, and some redirec-
tion. Starting in the early nineteenth century, it
took physics over 100 years to agree on what
statements about atoms meant. Now we take these
statements for granted. To agree on something, we
must first agree on a lot of other things. In everyday
commonsense realism, we humans agree on a taxonomy in which rocks sink in water, day differs
from night, and the sun is hot. In everyday life,
people are mainly very predictable in accordance
with rules and maxims of social behavior. Why
can't human scientists agree on their readings and
characterizations? A correct statement about interpretations is just as correct as one about electrons.

When I say described observations contain an
interpretive element, I must readily admit that
some facts are more refined than others. Some
readings derive more from us than from things in
the real world. Where and how to draw the line?

---

[6]See Ziman, J.: *Reliable Knowledge: An Exploration of the Grounds for Belief in Science* (London,
Cambridge University Press, 1978). A beautiful book despite its premature obituary for the
human sciences.

"Subjective" means the entire interpretation is personal; "objective" means it is intersubjective, semi-objective, public, human-centered and human-parametered. Even given masses of intersubjective, agreed-on facts, we can still wind up with more than one interpretation. Is light to be interpreted as a particle or a wave? Is physical space three-dimensional, four-dimensional, or *n*-dimensional?

Mind
Scientist:

In the human sciences, the initial hurdle lies in the descriptive characterization of intentional purposive action. Intentional action is a final output of mental activity, but there are many other processes leading up to it such as those involving affects. First, we must gain some degree of consensibility about actions. Human behavior is often described and explained in intentional, purposive, effectivity, goal-seeking terms. Clouds and rocks can be described and explained without a vocabulary of such terms because we do not attribute to clouds and rocks purposes and internally coded representations able to convert information into significances. Perhaps we should. But living-systems' behavior is understood by us in intentional terms.

Suppose ethologists see a bird flying across the sky. Is it migrating, is it escaping a predator, or is it foraging for food? You have to know lots more about the situation before you can gain consensus as to how to characterize what the bird is doing. Ethologists gain consensus that, for example, the bird is foraging because they know the animal well, have studied it for a long time in many different situations, and know what features are characteristic of foraging situations versus fleeing-predator situations. I see no good reason why, for example, agreement could not be reached in characterizing patients as having similar key idea

Psychiatric
Scientist:

profiles, as proposed by the Grantsman.

It might be that we fail to get agreements in the human sciences because of the level of the subject matter. We more easily get agreements about the human organism when we are close to the level of non-symbolic hardware (e.g. breathing rates and blood pressures that can be specified more precisely than, for example, beliefs whose contents are described in natural language). When we get to higher-level programs showing great flexibility and diversity of cultural content, agreements are harder to come by. The mind seems ill-at-ease in understanding itself and more-at-ease in understanding hardware. The terms of mental-functional descriptions are not in a one-to-one relation with their significance or meaning, nor even a many-to-one. The relations are many-to-many. In our society, the significance-semantic content of high-level programs are interwoven with our metaphysics and ideologies about, for example, issues of free will and determinism, mind and brain, people and machines. If I am to agree with you, I may have to change a long-standing ideological commitment about machines, which I am not about to give up easily.

And there is human perversity. People have to *want* to agree. People are competitive, combative, envious, truculent. Science is a communal enterprise and runs on consensus. But the first level of consensus is *taxonomic consensibility*, to use Ziman's term. We have to agree on what kinds exist or occur in the world before we can begin to count instances of kinds for inductive inferences. It is difficult to make progress at all in understanding our subject matter unless we can group our entities of inquiry into meaningful and distinct categories. When interpretations disagree, at least the interpreters must agree there is something independent the interpretations are *about*. Otherwise it is all a waste of time and other resources.

Inquirer:

Consensus means sufficient agreement, not necessarily unanimity. But what percentage of the expert community is "sufficient"? Five percent, 20 percent, 80 percent? This seems to be an overly authoritarian view of things. A statement affirmable as correct originates in a solitary individual and its acceptance as correct occurs ultimately in another solitary individual. If *you* say "X is true," how do I assure *myself* that X is true (i.e. truth$_2$)? Verification is a private matter of the individual. Every man must accept belief for himself, and there is no guaranteed escape from self-doubt and error. The whole world may agree but be wrong. Numerically, most of the people in the world still believe in witches. Members of the expert community have been educated, enjoined, and indoctrinated as youths to view the world in a certain way and hence they will tend to react loyally in a way similar to their colleagues. Consensus among experts may mean only that they have very similar nervous systems.

Mind
Scientist:

One reason scientific consensus is so impressive is that scientists themselves are argumentative, individualistic, and stubborn. If they tend to agree about their communications, whose recipients are enjoined to view reality in a certain way, then arguments and evidence of these messages must be persuasive enough and have sufficient rhetorical power to overcome the disputatious nature of scientists' personalities. Consensus can be achieved in a number of ways not all of which would lead to progress. Some are legitimate and some not. Political pressures, economic factors, colleagueship, simple submission to authority, and ideological conformity can generate consensus. Lysenko in Russia forced biologists to agree on his inheritance-of-acquired-characteristics view.

Biological
Scientist:

But only biologists in Russia agreed because that was where he had power. Being international, scientific judgment cannot be controlled by any one nation. Scientific consensus is free to the extent that it can be continuously challenged and tempered by criticism. Science does rest on authority in that not anyone can criticize its claims but only someone who is deemed competent in the field by other scientists.

Young
Psychiatrist:

We yield to authority in medicine and psychiatry. Psychoanalysts seem to have consensus that what Freud said is correct even though to some the ideas are uncompelling, if not just mystery mongering, in that psychoanalysts like to say what they think are dark things.

Clinical
Psychologist:

But psychoanalysis is only part of the relevant expert community. And if not challenged from within, it is certainly challenged from without. Other behavioral scientists are involved in these problems, and they do not agree about many psychoanalytic ideas. I, too, was at first bothered by the Metaphysician's claim that what we "see" are interpretations, but I now see he has a much larger view of what qualifies as an interpretation. Like my psychiatric colleagues, I have over the years listened to thousands of "expert" interpretations regarding patients. They often sounded like undergraduate exercises in English literature or biblical exegeses in which someone pontificates what a sentence in a text "really means." In clinical psychology, we gave up on Rorschach tests because the interpretations were simply too subjective.

Metaphysician:

It is not for me to poach and preach sermons on how to do research. All I can do is comment on the world views being utilized and perhaps recommend one over another as more suitable for the purposes of a particular field. I will stick to my position that we do not see a thing by itself. We see it is a thing of a certain kind (i.e. we construct an interpretation), what the Mind Scientist more precisely calls a *characterization*.[7]

Mind
Scientist:

We don't always have the right code to separate the message signs from the noise, to grasp which underlying patterns are best for us. If you don't want to call them *interpretations*, call them *readings* or *characterizations*. These kinds are our facts. I would call them significations since they involve signs bearing significance or meaning for interpreters. Significations may be the crucial invariants for the human sciences, because signs stand *for* something, they signify, and this significate is a meaning. Persons act in accordance with their situations and in accordance with rules they apply in these contexts.

Metaphysician:

If you are going to read the signs in the domain of mental disorders, conditions that people do *not* want, you are on the right metaphysical track of

---

[7]Interpretation assigns meaning to informational signs. Galileo used a book analogy: "Philosophy is written in that great book which forever lies before our eyes. I mean the universe. But we cannot understand it if we do not first learn the language and grasp the symbols in which it is written." See Galileo, G.: *The Assayer*. For Galileo, the signs, symbols, and language were those of mathematics, but by mathematics he meant circles and triangles. Mathematics is a language with many dialects. What sort of mathematics is most suitable for the problem?

Science searches for the best mathematical description whose formulae have well-understood properties. These properties can be manipulated in a theoretic-symbolic space, independent of their referents in the empirical problem space, and then mapped back onto these empirical referents, transformed, to see if this expedites a solution to the problem. Sometimes during the symbolic play with a mathematical formalism, we find something that we did not notice in studying the empirical system. When we return to the empirical problem, we may do so enriched with a mathematically derived surplus or bonus. The mathematical system applied may contain all kinds of elements and artifices not believed to be true for the empirical system. What sort of physical interpretation is to be given to $\sqrt{-1}$? Einstein sided with Galileo: "The really creative principle is in mathematics. In a certain sense I consider it therefore to be true — as was the dream of the Ancients that pure thought is capable of grasping reality." See Einstein, A.: *The World As I See It* (Covici Friede, 1934). Needless to say, the appropriate mathematical language and formalism in the human sciences are still not very well worked out.

pragmatic realism whether you call the facts interpretations or not. If our own representations are in
part autobiographical artifacts, other such works of
art might be analyzed to gain some insights. If you
realize you are dealing with signs, messages, interpretations and constructs, it might help the human
sciences to come into closer contact with other
sources of knowledge about the fine structure of
message content in persons, such as found in the
themes of history, literature, biography, drama, et
cetera. Max Frisch said that novels objectivize
human subjectivities.

Academic Clinician: I have heard this advice for years. Reading
history, biographies, et cetera is interesting, but
it has not increased useful knowledge about mental disorders. Ideas and themes in literature are
all well and good in their place. The Grantsman
finds key ideas in patient accounts, but this does
not tell us *why* a patient is so concerned with these
topics.

Grantsman: As I said previously, when you try to run before
you can walk, you get too far ahead of yourself.
Finding key ideas is the natural history, taxonomic phase of inquiry dealing with manifest
properties. Once you have some reliable taxonomic information, you can begin to formulate
hypotheses about underlying explanations. There
is no point in trying to explain why lightning
freezes wine if it does not do so. Explanatory
knowledge is dependent on prior taxonomic
knowledge.

Psychiatric Scientist: To constrain the proliferation of characterizations, we need more intersubjective, semi-
objective tests and methods. As Charles Peirce
maintained, it isn't just the facts, but the manner
in which you obtained them that counts. The
Grantsman is offering us a new method and a

new instrument, using a precise, more objective, and consistent computer algorithm, that restricts personal subjectivity. In developing such an alternative taxonomy, our problem is to find new kinds of phenomena, not to relate the kinds we already have. I think we have gleaned all the facts we can from standard clinical interviews. We need to insert new instruments between ourselves and the patient. I think the Grantsman's proposal is a good try, but to me it is too thin a reed on which to erect a whole classification system for mental illness. The Grantsman's method addresses itself to only one sort of properties, conceptual patterns and key ideas. As the Biological Scientist points out, several different sorts of properties are needed to build informationally rich taxonomies. Facts must fit other facts as well.

Grantsman: Since classes of complex objects are polythetic, with no two individuals necessarily sharing the same property, a large number of properties are needed.[8] It depends on the purposes of a field and the job a taxonomy is supposed to help us with. One kind of property may be sufficient for a particular job. For example, in medicine the single property of blood group is extremely useful for purposes of transfusion. What additional sorts of properties do you have in mind for a psychiatric classification?

Psychiatric
Scientist: Your description of your proposal has given me

---

[8]For the distinction between monothetic and polythetic classes, see Dialogue V, "The Biological Scientist." The concept of polythetic class thus denies there can be any essence to a class. Every member of a polythetic class need not share a particular property. (This does not imply, however, that he *must* not). The probability of an individual being a member of a polythetic class depends on how many of the properties defining the class he exhibits, and the properties can be weighted for degrees of relevance. This loose definition of a class is disconcerting to the traditionalist who insists on a strict conjunction of properties, but this open-disjoint way of looking at classes seems to be "the way it is," at least for now. The problem with such cluster classes is where to set the threshold of entry.

an expanded, and maybe too expansive or extravagant, idea. I would like to see designed a more comprehensive research project conducted somewhat as follows. Start with an initial collection of psychiatric complainants and non-complainant controls between the ages of 18 and 40 who are not brain-damaged, not in grossly psychotic states, not alcoholic, and not drug abusers. These are people who have been traditionally classified under the "neuroses," but the term and class is too vague to be useful. I am willing to let experienced clinicians decide that the subjects are *not* members of the groups specified to be excluded. They may miss once in a while, but you have to start someplace and not worry too much about sharply defining the initial collection of entities, as the Grantsman noted. The complainants are patients mentally dysfunctional in some way, whereas the controls are not. You use the controls for comparisons in the usual way.

I would then let the Grantsman find the key idea profiles and group individuals with similar profiles using a cluster analysis. To this information I would add at least four other sorts of properties: (a) overt behavioral, (b) psychophysiological, (c) psychological, and (d) neuropsychological. For example, McGuire and his associates have worked out methods of coding overt observable behavior of patients in naturalistic settings.[9] Let him also form groups using a cluster analysis with any measure of similarity he chooses as suited to his data. Follow the same process using psychophysiological measurements and also novel psychological tests.

Imagine a row-column matrix with each patient heading a column, each row representing a kind of property, and each cell containing the

---

[9]See McGuire, M. T., and Fairbanks, L. A. (Eds.): *Ethological Psychiatry: Psychopathology in the Context of Evolution Biology* (New York, Grune and Stratton, 1977).

the name of the group the patient is clustered in according to the four kinds of properties (draws on blackboard) (see Fig. 9). An analysis of this matrix shows, for example, that patients P_1, P_3, P_4 in Group IV ideationally also cluster in Group B_2 behaviorally, PP_5 psychophysiologically, and P_3 psychologically. Now you can form a superordinate polythetic group. At its initial baptism, let's call it Type I, in which the members share some proportion of three different sorts of properties. Each approach finds groups by correlations in its data matrix. Congruence of these groups with groups from other approaches is found by matrix correlations.[10]

PATIENTS

PROPERTY GROUPS	P_1	P_2	P_3	P_4	P_5	.....
IDEATIONAL	G_{IV}	G_{II}	G_{IV}	G_{IV}	G_{IV}	.....
BEHAVIORAL	B_2	B_1	B_2	B_2	B_6	.....
PSYCHO-PHYSIOLOGICAL	PP_5	PP_4	PP_5	PP_5	PP_5	.....
PSYCHOLOGICAL	P_3	P_1	P_3	P_3	P_3	.....

Figure 9. The Matrix of Patient Groups.

---

[10]The Psychiatric Scientist is describing an approach to psychiatric taxonomy alternative to that of the traditional system in which properties, rather than individuals, are grouped. Suppose the data matrix looked like this:

Properties			Individuals		
	1	2	3	-----	n
1	X_{11}	X_{12}	X_{13}		
2	X_{21}	X_{22}	X_{23}		
3	X_{31}	X_{32}	X_{34}		
,					
,					
,					
n					

The entry X_{11} means individual *1* has property *1*, etc. A Q technique groups the columns of individuals; an R technique groups rows of properties.

Grantsman: Hold it. Surely, this is too grandiose and over-optimistic. If things happen that way, we would be more than happy. What seems more likely is that you will have a lot of scatter and overlap. Perhaps members of one of my groups will not cluster at all in a way groups cluster in the other assessment components of the study.

Psychiatric
Scientist: That's possible, but there is only one way of finding out and that is to go ahead and try. As the famous engine inventor said, "Start her up and see why she don't go." Notice patient P_5 in the matrix. Although he fits the groups of patients P_1, P_3, and P_4, he does not cluster in the behavioral group B_2. Something is amiss, and there is work to be done. The investigators must reexamine the data on patient P_5. He may be an outlier in either cluster, and if we recluster him in ideational Group III, he may fall into behavioral Group B_6 or vice versa. Or he just doesn't fit anywhere too well.

                      The statistical analyses must be combined with clinical judgments as to what is relevant or important. A scientist makes his living by taking different things as similar; a statistican makes his by taking similar things as identical. Knowledge about the clinical domain must guide the statistical treatments of the data. The advantage of having such data is, as I have described, that we can reiterate through them again and again looking for new clusterings.

                      Another weakness of the current classification system is that it has no built-in systematic procedures like this for monitoring itself, recognizing mistakes, and self-correction. One has to keep working at a taxonomy and learn from successive appraisals and reappraisals.[11]

---

[11]As an early taxonomist said, taxonomy is a process of *tatonnement* or groping: de Candolle, 1816, quoted in Sneath and Sokal, *Numerical Taxonomy* p. 20. It is arrived at *a posteriori* by continuous empirical wrestling and struggle on the part of those willing to do so. Classifications become shaped and reshaped in the light of further experience and new information.

Old Psychiatrist:	You have talked about illness or patient groups with the individuals having similar properties. Do you mean the patients in these illness groups have the same mental disease or disorder?
Psychiatric Scientist:	I have said nothing about disease, disease entities, or disorder. Our first job is to group individual patients according to shared properties. We would not be classifying disease, but ill people. Ill people in the similarity classes would then be considered for similar management decisions.
Clinical Psychologist:	I have some qualms about the proposal as it now stands. You plan to collect data on five sets of variables — ideational, overt-behavioral, psychophysiological, psychological, and neuropsychological. Then you hope to find correlations or congruences between the groups based on these variables, members of a group based on one set of variables being also members of a group based on another set of variables. I can see the value of this sort of multiple convergence. To do all this you will need a large number of experimental and control subjects on whom you will collect a large amount of data. My first worry is you will wind up with the usual mountains of data that you will be unable to analyze in any meaningful way because you won't know what a clinically useful group is. How will you utilize clinical judgments about applicability? You may form groups, or even a superordinate type based on three subgroups, but how will you know you have anything worthwhile unless you further test the group for treatment response or prognosis?
Grantsman:	She is worried about two things. First is the standard problem of having too large a number of variables and of reducing dimensionality in a large set of dimensions that are not really independent. My guess would be that most of the initial variables will turn out to be irrelevant. Also many of them will be redundant and superfluous. Second, she is

suggesting that we must conduct a larger study to see if the groups, if some are found, have any clinical value such as predicting to some criterion. One should try to make predictions on a new sample of our reference population. Suppose we find that patients in ideational Group IV are congruent with the other property groups. Now knowing something about the composition or structure of the reference population, we can draw a new sample according to some sampling plan. In this sample, when we identify a patient as a member of ideational Group IV, we might predict how he will be clustered by the other components of the study with some probability p.[12]

If there is accord among samples coordinated by a similar sampling plan, we gain further assurance that we have a dependable cluster. This gives us some degree of predictive validity. Still, it does not answer the question as to the utility of the cluster for clinical purposes of management or treatment. We may have nice groups mathematically, as determined by the clustering algorithm, but are they useful? The properties on which we are basing the clusters might not be relevant to management decisions. Why not go ahead and give members of the cluster similar treatments or no-treatments? The outcomes of such management decisions would close the loop of a feedback cycle.

Psychiatric
Scientist: The feedback information might result in a revision of the original groups. That is, what combination of properties and absence of properties are shared by individuals having a similar response to a management decision? They may

---

[12]As has been discussed in previous dialogues, probabilities must be taken into consideration. Patient-states are probabilistic and our knowledge of them lacks certainty. One can rarely assert with near certainty (i.e. $p = 1.0$) what a future patient-state will be. A probability is a conjectured proportion about a future imagined world of many possible states, most of which never happen.

not correspond to the combinations of properties used in forming the initial clusterings. The re-groupings would provide the most useful information for the clinician, which is, after all, the purpose of a psychiatric taxonomy to begin with. This ability to revise the classification based on a publicly open testable data base that can be added to, and reiteratively worked over, I see as a major virtue of the proposed project.

Academic Clinician: Let us suppose such a research project were conducted. How does it differ from other projects, and what other advantages would it give us?

Psychiatric Scientist: The strategy of the project differs in the following ways:

(1) It is based on grouping individuals systematically found to be sharing measurable properties rather than being based on clinically intuited property sets of disease entities or their prototypes.

(2) It utilitizes numerous properties as well as different sorts of properties in addition to conventional signs and symptoms.

(3) It utilizes computer algorithms (a) in discovering ideational properties, (b) in forming groups (i.e. instead of relying on impressionistic correlations of clinicians), and (c) in creating machine-readable records for a data base.

(4) Using the machine-readable records, the system can be monitored over time, errors can be recognized, and self-corrections take place through fed-back experience regarding clinical utility — these being improvement strategies lacking in current classification systems.

(5) It constructs a multidimensional data base that is publicly available and scrutinizable, extensible, and iteratively testable to form

new groups based on new data from a variety of investigators.

Academic Clinician: So far so good and even impressive. But my second question was, what does it do for me? How will all this help the clinician who is trying to help the patient?

Psychiatric Scientist: If this alternative taxonomy works out, we would be able to make the following kinds of statements:

(1) Patients of Type IV with properties a and b and c or d, but not j, will show decreased symptoms of anxiety 86 percent of the time when given therapy T_1 under the following conditions. . . .

(2) Patients of Type IV with the same properties as in statement (1) will show an increase in symptoms of anxiety 20 percent of the time when given therapy T_2 under the following conditions. . . .

And so forth. The statements are useful to clinicians because they provide information on which he can base his future-oriented management decisions with individual patients. Clinicians will have more reliable predictive abilities.

Academic Clinician: I know it may sound strange to the rest of you, but in listening to this *I have changed my mind*. I am beginning to like this idea of having similarity groups of individuals who are candidates for similar management decisions. It liberates us from our strait-jacket of worry about what is *the* disease, *the* disorder or *the* diagnosis. Our concern should be the patient's multiple illness conditions and how to deal with them. Hence, I would be in favor of this taxonomic research project. Intuitively, clinicians know they are treating individual conditions rather than diseases. If successful, the research would be emancipatory for them and give them a new self-respect.

Old
Psychiatrist:

The proposal is getting out of hand. It involves numerous clinical and technical research experts, a support staff and a computer system. All these will involve considerable expense over a span of years. It smacks to me of big science which spends millions but benefits no one except those on the payroll. The rising costs of such inquiries may not be commensurate with the returns, even if there are any. And wouldn't the whole project have to be replicated by another research group of comparable composition using the same procedures?

Psychiatric
Scientist:

Not necessarily. Only parts of it need to be repeatable to assure the usefulness of the groups found. Suppose we find a superordinate group, Type I, whose members cluster on ideational behavioral, psychophysiological and psychological variables. Let's dream a little further and suppose 80 percent respond favorably to treatment X. In adding a new property to members of the group (i.e. treatment response), the group remains stable. Through this sort of retrovalidation, we can then raise our confidence that members of the group share properties, making the group a useful kind. New patients, say in another part of the country, could be identified as Type I using an identification key made up of a number of properties much smaller than those used in forming the original classification. Many properties are needed to establish a classificatory system. Once established, only a few properties are needed to assign an individual to the proper class. The properties might even be those of only one sort, say ideational.

If new patients respond favorably to treatment X at about 80 percent rate, then we have further evidence justifying the soundness of the Type I superordinate group. We could provisionally generalize that a patient of Type I will respond favorably to treatment X with a probability of 0.8. If a patient can be identified as a type using a key, the clinician will know, with some degree of probability, what property-states he must deal with because these are consequences of the patient being a member of this type, an inductive group. Some clinicians do not like probabilities applied to a single patient. Then we just tell him what proportion of similar patients responded favorably to treatment X and let him decide whether to use this information as a guideline in his own management decision.

Biological
Scientist: Your description stresses the important distinction we must keep in mind between classification (i.e. forming the initial clusters) and identification (i.e. ascertaining whether a new entity belongs to a cluster already formed using a key). Before anyone asks how a key is constructed, let me say the methods for constructing keys are fully explained in Sneath and Sokal.[13]

Grantsman: I agree the proposal is an improvement over mine because of the increased information and cross-referencing obtained from using different sorts of properties. Now there are additional realities to be considered. Several of you here have said that reality contains objects which object and one thereby becomes stuck. Many of our objects in the world are other people. A current research obstacle is the great difficulty in obtaining funds to support innovative research in which something is done for the first time and the outcome is unpredictable. What funding agencies want is a brand new idea that has been thoroughly tested and found to be successful

[13]See Sneath and Sokal, *Numerical Taxonomy* (p. 382).

before they will begin to support it. To obtain findings, one must first obtain new fundings. It is not just the resistance of the problem we must overcome but also the resistance to giving out money for exploratory research. The main constraint on scientific progress in the 1980s is economic, not conceptual. There is no lack of good ideas.

Old
Psychiatrist:

Surely, millions of dollars a year are poured into mental health research. And from the practitioners' perspective, we have very little to show for it. In the cost-benefit sense, most clinical research has been a waste of the taxpayers' money. Perhaps it should be decelerated or curtailed and the money used for something else, like improving hospital care.

Young
Psychiatrist:

In fact, most of the discoveries in psychiatry of the past 30 years have been lucky accidents. The story goes that in 1948 an Australian psychiatrist, believing that manic psychosis was a biochemical disturbance, tested the effect of uric acid from manic patients on guinea pigs. Uric acid salts are not very soluble. So he tried lithium urate on one group of guinea pigs and used lithium carbonate on another group for control of the effects of lithium. When both groups of animals became lethargic, he tried lithium on manic patients, all of whom improved clinically. Now lithium carbonate is one of our chief medications for manic excitement.[14]

Biological
Scientist:

But the psychiatrist was *looking*; he was *after* something. Some sort of systematic search was being conducted. Luck is the residue of design. It

---

[14]The psychiatrist was John Cade. It was ten years before his discovery was adopted because lithium is cheap in contrast to other psychotropic drugs whose promotional campaigns bring millions of dollars into the pharmaceutical industry. See Beveridge, W.I.B.: *Seeds of Discovery* (New York, Norton, 1980, p. 39). For historical buffs, the original reference is Cade, J.F.J.: Lithium salts in the treatment of psychotic excitement (*The Medical Journal of Australia*, 36:349, 1949).

is often said that the discovery of penicillin in 1928 was accidental because the spores blew into Fleming's laboratory through an open window. But Fleming was looking for something that destroyed bacteria. If you carry it far enough, every happening is riddled with chains and intersections of accidental events. Fleming chose to work at this old hospital, in preference to a more prestigious one, because he liked to swim and the old hospital had a swimming pool. [15]

Billions, not millions, have been poured into cancer research with only a few helpful results. You have to pile up masses of diverse evidence and mutually corroborating facts. Mendeleyev constructed the periodic table in chemistry using sixty-three elements. He could not have done it with three. By the way, it might interest psychiatrists that he began his classification with lithium.

I have a few final caveats for your quest. I would not suggest we give up cancer or mental illness research. These are among the scourges of mankind. Mental illness is a massive and primary health problem. It represents a highly intractable problem in which it is as difficult to produce a third magnitude result as it is to produce a first magnitude result in other domains. As in diving contests at swimming meets, a degree of

---

[15]There are several versions of the charming Fleming penicillin story. Some say the old hospital offered Fleming a job because they wanted him both on their rifle team and water-polo team. Others say the old window neither opened nor closed properly. Still others claim the spores came up the stairwell from a downstairs laboratory where research on molds was being conducted. A remarkable point is that bacteriologists in the nineteenth century, including Pasteur, knew that molds of the *Penicillium* family were antagonistic to the growth of bacteria. In 1897, a French medical student, Ernest Duchesne, even demonstrated in his dissertation research that penicillin was a successful antibiotic in animals. He suggested it might be used for the treatment of infectious diseases in humans. Nobody responded. It took World War II to push the story to its successful end. See Hare, R.: *The Birth of Penicillin* (London, Allen and Unwin, 1970). For Fleming's own version, see the interview with him by Jones, G.: *In The New Scientist* (May, 1981).

difficulty as well as how well the dive is performed must be considered in the final score. Incidentally, cancer research shares with mental illness research the problem of finding new properties. More pieces of the complex puzzle are needed. What unknown properties of cancer cells allows them to multiply, invade, and metastasize? The amount of money spent on research reflects a society's values. I used to say we spend more on chewing gum than on cancer research. I was understating the case. It turns out we spend more on just bubble gum, over one billion dollars per year in the United States, than we do on cancer research.

Research goes in cycles of fads and fashions like art and hair styles. Science can be viewed as the *uncovering* of truths. Failures are instructive. Perhaps psychiatry is not making its scientific mistakes fast enough.[16] Your reseach community is not yet large enough to generate a plurality of facts and theories. In my view, your field has not been sufficiently self-critical. And it may have methodological shibboleths. I gather it has not been fashionable to study the classification system in psychiatry. There have been objections to the crude botanization of patients and pigeonholing people.

Grantsman: For many years academic psychiatry was dominated by the psychoanalytic paradigm, a reaction to the Kraepelinian paradigm that diagnosed or labeled the patient and then did not do much to help him. Rightly so, psychoanalytic psychiatrists tried to understand what was wrong with the patient and tried to help him at the symbolic-mediational level with psychotherapeutic interventions. Attempts to ad-

---

[16]To have good ideas, one has to have lots of ideas, most of which are bad. In his later years, Einstein was asked if he noticed any change in his thought processes as he became older. He replied, "Yes, it takes me longer now to reject a bad idea."

dress the diagnosis problem were viewed as regressive, static, do-nothing, and empty labeling. But the current generation is beginning to realize how fundamental the diagnosis problem is for both clinical and research purposes. Not a month goes by now without a paper on diagnosis in some major psychiatric journal.

A lot of the money spent for mental illness research has been wasted due to the simple methodological error of having such heterogeneous samples of patients that no sense could be made out of the results. For every finding there was a contradictory finding. No matter how good your independent variable is, if your dependent variable — a bunch of patients — is sloppily formed, the outcome of the study will be dubious. Some mental health Potomacs realize this, but it is a difficult pill for them to swallow because it implies they have been going about it in the wrong way for a long time. Maybe it is fortunate that things are going so slowly in psychiatry because they are going in the wrong direction anyway. A proposal as described by the Psychiatric Scientist would not be well-received; it excites ill will.

Young
Psychiatrist: Who are the mental-health Potomacs?

. Grantsman: The government people in Washington who give out the money for research. Policy decision-makers and their staffs decide what research gets done and what does not get done — an awesome responsibility requiring a thick skin as well as courage. They tend to play it safe and continue doing what has been done. They also look after their buddies. Some in positions of power become swelled with the idea that they are steering the research of an entire nation. They arrogantly believe that if only the researchers were as smart as they are and would do things right, the problems would be solved. But some of the greatest minds of our time, like Pauling and Szent-Gyorgi, cannot get federal funding.

Government people are cautious and conservative. Like the rest of us, they want to keep their jobs. If they do so for too long, the imagination becomes dulled. The Potomacs' usual question is "How do you *know* it is going to work?" To me, research, by definition, means the outcome is unpredictable. Research is a process of going up alleys to see if they are blind. The Feds avoid the Type I error of backing and, hence, being responsible for a potential loser; in the meantime, they commit the Type II error of missing a potential winner. Most of the time they get losers anyway. They have forgotten that we do not only wish to avoid error but also to encompass truth. And they are vulnerable to Type III error of pouring money into trying solve the wrong problems, such as whether psychotherapy is effective.

Young Psychiatrist:	What's the matter with solving that problem?
Grantsman:	It is like asking if surgery is effective. *What* surgery, and the surgery of *what*? Is there evidence that neurosurgery is sufficiently effective to justify remuneration? If we cannot answer the taxonomic question of what *kinds* of patients are being treated, let alone by what *kind* of psychotherapy, how can this be taken seriously as a scientific question? The question sounds more political than anything else because of third-party payments for mental illness by insurance plans. There are many skin diseases, for example, for which there is no effective treatment. Does this mean patients should not consult dermatologists and receive treatment? Will insurance companies refuse to pay dermatologists for their attempts to treat psoriasis? Now the question becomes moral as well as political. The mentally ill and their helpers are always at the bottom of the heap.

Regardless of the findings of a study, bureaucrats will use them to serve their own interests and beliefs about mental illness.

Old
Psychiatrist: It must be difficult to criticize those on whom your research is totally dependent. Research is not a self-supporting enterprise. You are dependent on other people's money. You are biting the hand that might feed you. Aren't you afraid that by talking this way you will never get another grant? You and the Feds should be working together as partners for the common good and here the two of you are at odds. Do you really expect to hector, persuade, or goad government people into sponsoring your grant proposal?

Grantsman: No, not under the current regime, which is locked into backing DSM-III, an enterprise that has already become a gold mine for the profession. Planck said you simply have to wait for the entrenched opponents to die off. In the meantime, unfortunately, one can become dead oneself. We all know the federal mental health grant system is a paralyzed mess. Only 5-10 percent of proposals are funded. So 90-95 percent of investigators are frustrated and demoralized. They spend more time writing proposals than doing actual research. The mental health grant system needs a complete overhaul and some new blood.

Inquirer: But I thought the system relied on peer reviews. It is your peer colleagues who are rejecting the proposals, not the federals.

Psychiatric
Scientist: The Grantsman may have equals but he has no peers. A creative thinker puts the established world at risk. A peer review can be a sneer review. A peer reviewer is often a competitor who wants the funds for his own projects or for the school of thought he represents. In Britain, they call it the "old-boy" network. The Potomacs can select the peer

reviewers according to their own inclinations. They can stack the deck through judicious selection. And when peer reviewers make judgments sitting face-to-face around a table, the stronger personalities tend to win out. Proposals should be read and evaluated by reviewers without a committee meeting. Also, a grant should be given to an investigator, not to a proposal. I would fund people like Pauling and Szent-Gyorgi just on the basis of who they are as generators of bright ideas and what they have already accomplished.

Grantsman: You are still faced with the problem of a starting investigator who has no track record. His proposal must be evaluated. Also, I would suggest the grant proposer should be allowed to rebut negative judgments before a final decision is made. Nowadays, including a rebuttal in a resubmission of the proposal delays things for nine to twelve months, and the "peers" reviewing the new proposal may be an entirely different group of people who do not share the views of the initial peer group that recommended changes. The second peer group may say "why don't you do it *this* way," which was the way initially proposed to the first peer group. But enough wailing about our hardships. Every embittered investigator tends to equate the rejection of his grant proposals with the persecution of Galileo. We have been harping on the need for new factual knowledge.

In addition, the Psychiatric and Mind Scientists and myself are proposing a new perspective, a new way of looking at the facts and the problems of mental illness in terms of interferences with proper computational functions. Treatment would be conceptualized as attempting to emancipate the patient from restrictions on, or impairments in, his computational abilities. We are suggesting a fundamental change of mind about how the mind in general works. I would be interested in what the others have to say about our enjoinments to look at it this way.

Old
Psychiatrist: It is hard for me to evaluate it because I must confess ignorance about computers. I realize computers are here to stay, and they are all over the place these days. When a man has a hammer, everything looks like a nail. I have no objections to machine-readable records because I can see how they would improve our productivity and efficiency. Nor do I object to computers used for statistical data analysis or clustering groups in a taxonomy. It is when our minds are compared to computers that I balk. At best, a computer seems to be a glib and pop metaphor of the mind. My question is, is it a metaphor fruitful in consequences for psychiatry? Whether the fleshed-out metaphor can aid in solving our problems remains to be seen.

Mind
Scientist: The computer has become more than a metaphor. In a metaphor we deem two things to be similar or analagous in some respect. We say, for example, "a man is a wolf" with an implied similarity along a dimension of say "ferocity." An equivalence class is more than a metaphor because it comprises a *contagious* analogy in which the similarity relation is transitive such that given the members of the class a, b, c, d we also can say "a is like b, b is like c, and thus c is like d." In the man-wolf metaphor, we don't say "man is like a wolf, a wolf is like a dog, and thus man is like a dog." In certain respects, as symbol-matter systems, people and computers are members of an equivalence class, a relation much stronger than metaphoric.

Academic
Clinician: I am not an infuriated humanist, but also I am not enthralled by peddlers of paradigms in which people are compared to machines. People are even advocating computer psychotherapy.[17]

---

[17]See Colby, K. M.: Computer psychotherapists. In Sidowski, J. B., Johnson, J. J., and Williams, T. A. (Eds.): *Technology in Mental Health Care Delivery Systems* (New Jersey, Ablex, 1980, p. 109).

I hear that computer therapy for depression is already underway.

Psychiatric
Scientist:

One reason psychiatry is so backward is that it resists modern technology, both high and low. It is still mainly pretechnological. Where I work, it took me five years to convince the authorities to get a Xerox photocopying machine, and we still don't have a word-processor. We need physical as well as conceptual tools. The thought of a computer doing something other than payrolls horrifies many established psychiatrists. They did psychiatry without a computer, so why should you need one? Record-keeping has always been done by hand; machine-readable records to them are a mere frill and a passing fad.

Academic
Clinician:

We have enough ways of dehumanizing people without adding another one such as comparing them to a computer. The purpose of a field like psychiatry is to help people by reducing their mental suffering. Machines don't suffer; they do not feel.

Mind
Scientist:

A subtle but powerful point. You suggest a disanalogy which, at one stroke, might wipe out the positive analogy between minds and computers so appealing to the Psychiatric Scientist, the Grantsman, and myself. The issue of awareness and L-consciousness in computers came up between the Inquirer and myself.[18] No one jumped on it the way I thought they would until now. Does a computer experience suffering when it does not do what it is designed to do? Being miserable may not characterize a computer going wrong. Artificial coloring is a color, but an artificial flower is not a flower.

Here we must *very carefully* differentiate using a computer as a model to represent something, in contrast to making it into a literal replica, a com-

---

[18]See Dialogue VI, p. 103.

plete duplicate, or a clone of the real thing. A computer *model* of a hurricane is not itself wet. You feed it descriptions and you get back descriptions, none of which are even moist. A computer program consists of strings of symbols. It can have symbolic representations of affect that act on other kinds of representations. The model does not "have," say, enjoyment any more than a differential equation may have a symbolic representation of radioactivity but is not itself radioactive. A computer does not suffer; we *represent* suffering in a program symbolically. Whether future computers will suffer may ultimately depend on what the system is made of. If it consists of wires and silicon transistors, we doubt if it suffers. But if this "machine" were made of living cells, would we believe that it suffers if it says so and gives other indications of sufferings we impute to a living system? Perhaps then we would not call it a machine at all, but a man-made organism. But is it an animal or a plant? Do plants suffer? The computational paradigm works with the concept of a "virtual machine." That is, it is not concerned with what stuff the machine is physically made of, only with its computational functions and abilities.

Psychiatric
Scientist: To me, a computer is not a machine at all. It is merely laboratory jargon to call it a machine. A computer system is an instrument like a violin or a piano on which all kinds of music can be played. We shouldn't confuse the music with the instrument. Music is the software. Think of software as what can be sent over a phone line. You can't send a piano over a phone line.[19] It is not computers per se that we three here are interested in; it is their software programs and what they

_____

[19]This concrete analogy to help the uninitiated understand computers is proposed by Hofstadter, *Gödel, Escher, Bach* (p. 302)

can do that is important. More precisely, it is not what computers can do but what can they be *made* to do. What can a pencil do? It can be made to write novels, draw pictures, do arithmetic.

One can view computers and their programs as constituting a *special kind* of machine, one we in our evolutionary process have made in our own mental image. Growing up around this instrument and its programs is a body of concepts, assumptions, characterizations, interpretations and significations that may take psychiatry a long time to digest, especially when it is still struggling to accept word-processors. It took medicine 300 years to accept the concept of vitamins. Leading nineteenth-century physicists, such as Faraday, Mach, and Ostwald, refused to accept the existence of atoms. Great men should be allowed a few mistakes.

The computational paradigm provides a new stratum of conceived reality to investigate, a new range of possibilities. In addition to the physical, chemical, and biological property-states of a system, we posit symbolic-representational property-states. New research strategies will be needed to explore the patterns and range of possibilities within the laminae of this symbol stratum of reality. People have proper computational capacities designed to be in good working order. Certain diminutions or interferences with these capacities characterize classes of people with mental illness. At least this view points to public mechanisms which can become part of objective, intersubjectively testable knowledge. Psychiatry, like medicine, has a compassionate Samaritan function in attempting to help, to comfort, to give information, to restore peace of mind. But it also has a responsibility to utilize the best scientific and technological knowledge of the time to fulfill its Samaritan function.

Old
Psychiatrist: But thus far, the computational paradigm has not

Inquirer:

helped a single psychiatric patient that I know of. That is what Harvey's contemporaries said about his view of the heart as a pump circulating blood. Disgusted by this shortsighted confusion of technical progress with conceptual innovation, he quit his research and became the royal physician. We must wait with forbearance and give a new perspective a grace period. It may well be that viewing our problems in terms of hardware and programs and all their consequences may not be fruitful. If no one works on it, nothing will get done — a tautology, but some tautologies are more instructive than others.

Biological Scientist:

My one objection to the computational view is that it has been overly dominated by mathematical deductivism. Most computer scientists grow up in a Euclidean mathematical tradition in which everything is explained like geometry by deducing consequences from a few axioms taken as self-evidently true. But in the factual sciences, we start from hypotheses that are simply plausible conjectures and connect them, not just by deduction, with empirical generalizations. We do not know if the starting premises are true. Even if they were, one can come to false conclusions from true premises because one does not have all the required premises. In dealing with living systems, it is insufficient to view them in straightforward, linear, chugging-ahead, theorem-proving terms. Organisms represent highly interconnected, cyclic, circular, and web-like systems whose subsystems are reciprocally supportive. The workings of the brain affect the workings of the heart and vice versa. Artificial intelligence is weak on the empirical generalization side of things. If artificial intelligence is going to contribute to our knowledge of mental processes, it will have to free itself from a narrow deductive view and adopt the method of both logical and empirical approximations used in the factual sciences.

Mind
Scientist:

For me, deducible does not necessarily mean "deductive" in the strict sense of classical logic. It can mean "inferrable," "derivable," or even "computable." Everybody wants you to be like them. Mathematicians want us to specify probabilities, biologists want us to write programs that behave like organisms, physicians want us to write diagnostic programs which reason the way they think they do. But I agree with the Biological Scientist and her criticism. It bears on what has been said about finding the appropriate mathematical description. If our algorithms are to represent mental activity, they should function more like organisms do in being self-aware and self-correcting. I believe the future of artificial intelligence, as theoretical psychology, lies in the direction of constructing purposive, dynamic, multi-level, self-aware, and self-intervening systems. Thus far, most AI models have been flattened out, one-level systems with a slave mentality following the programmer's purposes rather than ones of their own.

Metaphysician:

I was struck by the point regarding the Samaritan function of psychiatry. It has already been noted that scientists repeatedly use affective terms such as *satisfying* and *satisficing*. I will entrust you with the little-discussed idea that science itself it ultimately affective in its aims. It enriches human life. I personally feel my life is enhanced by books, automobiles, television, and being able to play chess in my own room against the ingenious moves made by chess-playing computers. Science is supported by society because it gets people what they want and gets rid of what they do not want. Science is of human value in that it provides affectively advantageous knowledge, which helps people make rational choices with serious problems of ordinary life. For example, if my child is ill and perhaps dying, what course should I pursue? I should consult a medical expert whose knowledge derives from work in the medical sciences.

Science does not search just for knowledge and truths but for *valuable* knowledge and truths that enable us to make more rational choices with outcomes that are successful in affectively satisfying us as humans. I say this not to flatter people whose professions focus on affect as one of its crucial variables, but because I believe it to be true that science ultimately serves man's practical purposes of satisfying affective life. And if you think about it long enough. I think you will agree with me. Without this sort of affectively based social support, there would be no one around even to celebrate the scientists' predictions.

Inquirer: Our time is up. I hope everyone has had his say.[20]

---

[20]The group disperses. Speaking of affect, no one seems very satisfied about it all. Have they exhausted the subject, or vice versa? When all is said and done, more is said than done.

NAME INDEX

SUBJECT INDEX

229